A Practical Handbook of
PATHOLOGY
Specimens and Slides

A Practical Handbook of PATHOLOGY Specimens and Slides

Prithwiraj Maiti
RG Kar Medical College
Kolkata, West Bengal, India

JAYPEE The Health Sciences Publishers
New Delhi | London | Philadelphia | Panama

Jaypee Brothers Medical Publishers (P) Ltd

Jaypee Brothers Medical Publishers (P) Ltd
4838/24, Ansari Road, Daryaganj
New Delhi 110 002, India
Phone: +91-11-43574357
Fax: +91-11-43574314
Email: jaypee@jaypeebrothers.com

Overseas Offices

J.P. Medical Ltd
83 Victoria Street, London
SW1H 0HW (UK)
Phone: +44 20 3170 8910
Fax: +44 (0)20 3008 6180
Email: info@jpmedpub.com

Jaypee-Highlights Medical Publishers Inc
City of Knowledge, Bld. 237, Clayton
Panama City, Panama
Phone: +1 507-301-0496
Fax: +1 507-301-0499
Email: cservice@jphmedical.com

Jaypee Medical Inc
The Bourse
111 South Independence Mall East
Suite 835, Philadelphia, PA 19106, USA
Phone: +1 267-519-9789
Email: jpmed.us@gmail.com

Jaypee Brothers Medical Publishers (P) Ltd
17/1-B Babar Road, Block-B, Shaymali
Mohammadpur, Dhaka-1207
Bangladesh
Mobile: +08801912003485
Email: jaypeedhaka@gmail.com

Jaypee Brothers Medical Publishers (P) Ltd
Bhotahity, Kathmandu, Nepal
Phone: +977-9741283608
Email: kathmandu@jaypeebrothers.com

Website: www.jaypeebrothers.com
Website: www.jaypeedigital.com

Inquiries for bulk sales may be solicited at: jaypee@jaypeebrothers.com

A Practical Handbook of Pathology: Specimens and Slides

First Edition: 2014

Second Edition: 2023

Reprint 2024

ISBN 978-93-5152-414-4

Printed at:Replika Press Pvt. Ltd.

Dedicated to

All my juniors

Preface

The 2nd Professional MBBS examination is tough as it comes with a very wide syllabus, which a yet-newcomer medical student has to cover in a short time. For the pathology part, the systemic pathology remains an area of fear for many students as it looks lengthy and actually it is. The idea of this book came from this point.

It is a common fact everywhere that the questions asked in the Pathology Grand Viva actually start from the specimens and many students, even after reading their textbooks for 3 to 4 times remain very afraid of what questions will actually be asked. This book has covered a huge portion of systemic pathology and I think it will be helpful both for your theory as well as viva examinations. This book is not a textbook, but a supplement to textbooks.

As I am only in my Final Year MBBS and have a lot of things still unknown to me, I request everyone for any kind of feedback about this book. Please email me at prithwiraj2009@yahoo.in for any suggestions, queries or recommendations. I think this book will be a true companion of you at examination times. Thank you.

Prithwiraj Maiti

Acknowledgments

At the very beginning, I want to thank my parents, who have loved me always and have inspired me every moment to do something new. For the most of the photographs are taken by my friends Suvadeep Mandal and Debojyoti Dutta, the picture courtesy goes to them. I also want to thank my friends Suman Mandal and Bhaskar Roychoudhury for always staying with me and giving continuous support. My heartfelt thanks goes to all the staff of Jaypee Brothers Medical Publishers (P) Ltd family for working days and night to make this book a beautiful one especially to Shri Jitendar P Vij (Group Chairman), Mr Ankit Vij (Group President) and Mr Tarun Duneja (Director–Publishing) of M/s Jaypee Brothers Medical Publishers (P) Ltd, New Delhi, India, for publishing this book. I especially want to thank Mr Sabyasachi Hazra for his efforts towards publishing this 1st edition. At the end, the support from all my juniors is worth mentioning, because without their suggestions and feedbacks, it would be impossible to improvise the contents of this book. They have done the tough job of criticizing, which was also a main reason of student-friendliness of this book. Last but not least, it is worthy to mention those renowned pathologists and doctors who have accepted contributing their beautiful photographs in this book.

- *Dr Michael Danciu, MD, Pathologist Doctor of Medical Sciences, Lecturer Discipline of Pathology, University of Medicine and Pharmacy "Gr T Popa".*
- *Dr Frank Gaillard, Radiology Consultant at Royal Melbourne Hospital; Founder, Editor and CEO at Radiopaedia.org.*
- *Joel K Greenson, MD, Professor, Department of Pathology, University of Michigan.*
- *Allen Patrick Burke, MD, Pathologist, University of Maryland School of Medicine.*
- *Department of Clinical Laboratory Sciences, University of Cape Town, South Africa.*
- *Dr Ramaswami, MD, Nephrologist, Quensland, Australia.*
- *Dr Ed Uthman, MD, Clinical Pathologist and Anatomic Pathologist, Texas.*
- *Korean Endocrine Society.*
- *Dr Byung Joon Kim, Division of Endocrinology and Metabolism, Department of Internal Medicine, Konyang University College of Medicine, Korea.*
- *Rajkumar Elanjeran, Intern Doctor, Gandhi Medical College, Hyderabad.*
- *Dr Sajoscha Sorrentino, MD, Radiology Fellow, Hannover Medical School, Germany.*
- *Dr Jeremy Jones, MBChB MRCP FRCR PGDipMedEd, Radiology Fellow, Royal Children's Hospital, Melbourne, Australia.*
- *Health, Medicine, and Anatomy Reference Pictures.*
- *Dr Wael Nemattalla, Radiology Consultant, Suez Canal University Hospital, Egypt.*
- *Martha L Warnock, University of California, San Francisco.*
- *Dr Andrew Ryan, MD, Orthopedic Surgeon.*
- *Dr Charlotte L Ownby, Professor, Oklahoma State University College of Veterinary Medicine.*

Contents

SECTION–I

SPECIMENS

CHAPTER

1

Cardiovascular System

Mitral stenosis

Description

- It is a specimen of heart cut transversely.
- The left ventricle is recognized by its thick wall.
- The valve is lying between left ventricle and left atrium and having 2 cusps. So it is **mitral valve**.
- The valve has become thickened and fibrosed.
- The orifices have become grossly narrowed.
  - So, the specimen is identified as "Mitral stenosis" (Fig. 1.1).

What do you mean by stenosis?

Stenosis is the failure of a valve to open completely, which impedes forward flow (Fig. 1.2).

What do you mean by regurgitation/ insufficiency?

Regurgitation is the failure of a valve to close completely, thereby allowing reversed flow.

What is the major cause of mitral stenosis?

The major cause of mitral stenosis in India is chronic rheumatic heart disease.

Which age group is mostly affected?

School children (5–15 years age group).

What is the causative agent of rheumatic fever (RF) and rheumatic heart disease (RHD)?

- **RF is a delayed autoimmune response to Group A streptococcal pharyngitis.**

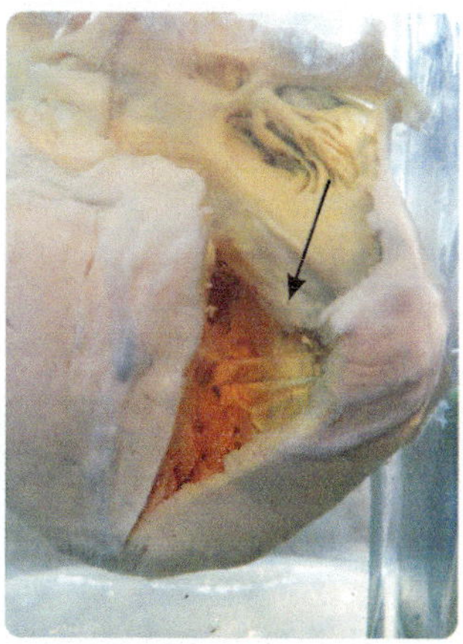

Fig. 1.1: Mitral stenosis. Specimen of heart, cut open to show cusps of mitral valve, which are thickened (arrow) and the opening is narrowed

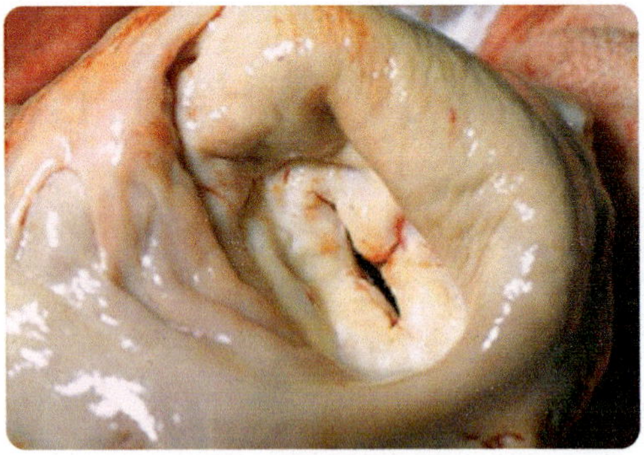

Fig. 1.2: Autopsy specimen showing thickened mitral valve leaflets with marked stenosis. Reproduced under the permission of Dr Jeremy Jones and Radiopaedia.org

- The clinical manifestations and severity of the disease depends on:
  1. Genetic susceptibility of the host
  2. Virulence of the infecting organism
  3. A favorable environment.
- Although streptococci from serogroups B, C, G, and F can cause pharyngitis, they are not linked to the etiology of RF or RHD.

Describe the pathogenesis of RF/ RHD.

- *Acute rheumatic fever (ARF) results from delayed immune responses to group A streptococcal antigens.*
- *Antibodies directed against the M-proteins of streptococci have been shown to cross-react with self-antigens in the heart.*
- In addition, *CD4+ T cells specific for streptococcal peptides* react with self-proteins of the heart and produce cytokines that activate macrophages and damage heart tissue.
- So, the damage to the heart tissue is thought to be caused by a *combination of antibody and T cell-mediated reactions.*
- The actual sequential events in the pathogenesis of RF/RHD is shown in Figure 1.3.

Note: Acute rheumatic fever never causes mitral stenosis in its first episode; but it may occur during recurrence and reactivation of the organism.

What is the role of streptococcal "M-protein" in the pathogenesis of RHD?

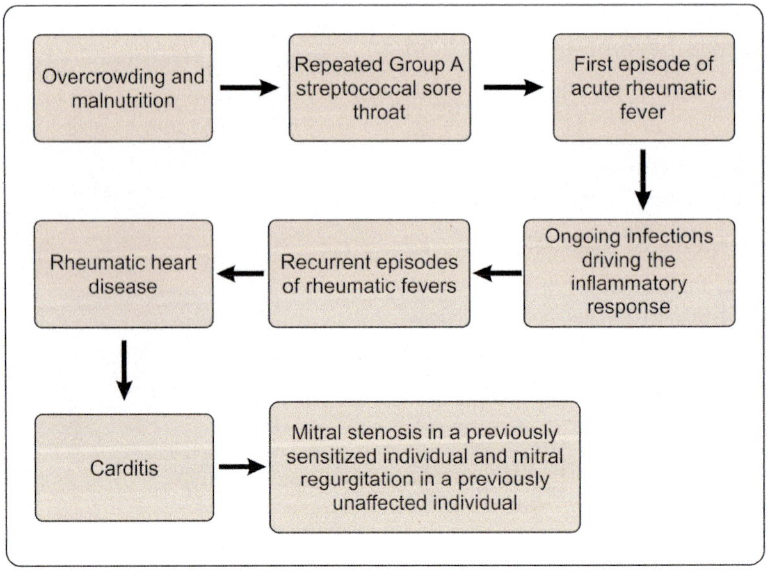

Fig. 1.3: Pathogenesis of mitral stenosis in RF/RHD

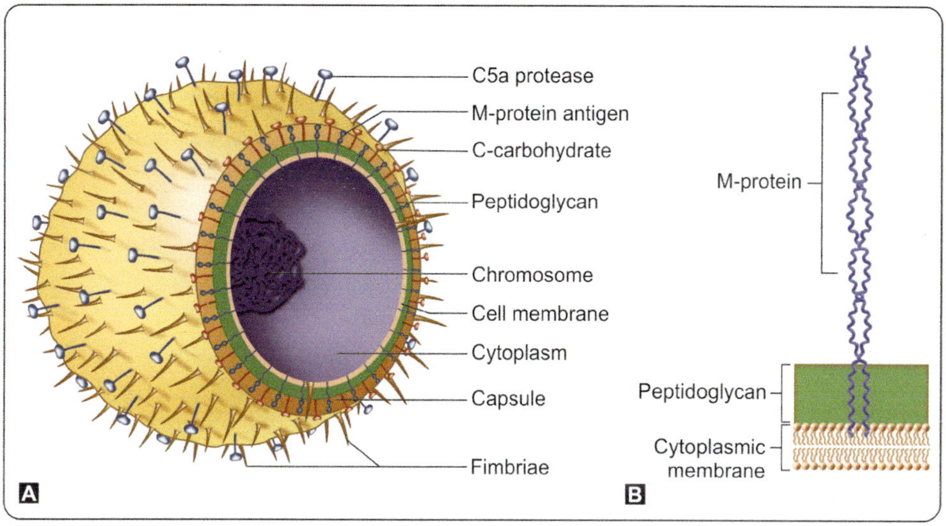

Figs 1.4A and B: A. Structure of a streptococcal cell, B. M-protein and its extension

- M-protein is one of the best-defined determinants of bacterial virulence in RHD.
- *The streptococcal M-protein extends from the surface of the cell as an alpha-helical coiled dimer (Figs 1.4A and B), and shares structural homology with cardiac proteins (myosin, tropomyosin and laminin); which are integral part of the cardiac valve and myocardium.*
  - It has been suggested that this homology is responsible for the characteristic pathological findings in acute rheumatic carditis.

What is the "toxic immunological hypothesis" of RF and RHD?

This hypothesis states that *some components of Group A streptococci have antigenic cross-relationship with human tissues* which is mostly responsible for their reaction against self-tissue antigens and also for the characteristic clinical manifestations found in RF/RHD.

What are the cardinal anatomic changes in the mitral valve?

1. Leaflet thickening
2. Commissural fusion and shortening
3. Thickening and fusion of tendinous cords.

Bacterial components	*Cross antigenic reaction against which host tissue?*
Capsule hyaluronic acid	Human synovial fluid and myocardium
Group A carbo-hydrate	Heart valve
M protein	Heart valve and myocardium
Cytoplasmic membrane	Vascular lamina
Peptidoglycan	Skin

What will be the microscopic appearance of the mitral valve?

Microscopically, the changes found in the mitral leaflets are:

1. Acute inflammation
2. Diffuse fibrosis
3. Neovascularization (new blood vessels formation).
   - This will eventually obliterate and destroy the leaflet architecture.

Questions about 'Aschoff body'

What is an 'Aschoff body'?

Aschoff bodies are pathognomonic lesions of rheumatic heart disease, characterized by presence of nodules in the heart resulting from inflammation of the heart tissue (Fig. 1.5).

Where they are predominantly found?

Usually in the myocardium and endocardium, in the vicinity of small blood vessels.

What is their microscopic appearance?

Microscopically, Aschoff body contains the following:

1. Anitschkow/Caterpillar cells: Activated macrophages characterized by linear condensations of nuclear chromatin (Fig. 1.6).
2. Foci of T-lymphocytes.
3. Necrosed collagen fibers.

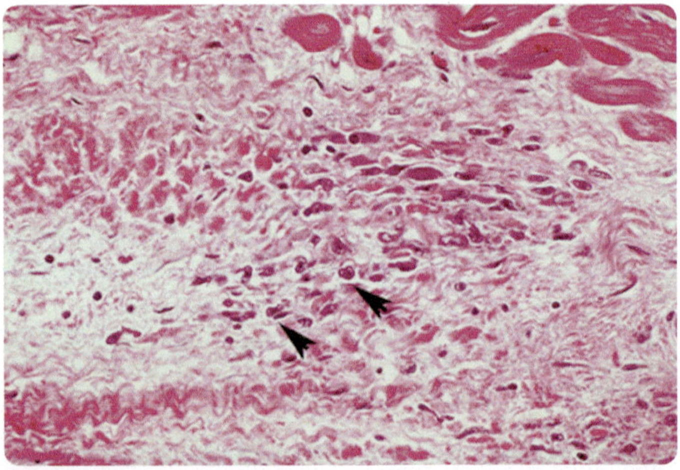

Fig. 1.5: Aschoff bodies (arrow heads): An interstitial aggregate of macrophages and lymphocytes with areas of fibrosis. Image reprinted with permission from Allen Patrick Burke, MD, University of Maryland School of Medicine, published by Medscape Reference (emedicine.medscape.com; 2013, available at: emedicine.medscape.com/article/1962779-overview)

What are the stages of evolution of Aschoff bodies?

Time of illness	Name of the stage	Characteristic features of the stage
4th week	Early exudative stage	• Edema of connective tissue • Increase in ground substance • Separation and eventual fragmentation of collagen fibers

Contd...

Contd...

Time of illness	*Name of the stage*	*Characteristic features of the stage*
		• Staining of the area characteristic of fibrin (fibrinoid necrosis)
4th–13th week	Intermediate proliferative stage	This is the stage of Aschoff bodies, characterized by presence of: • Anitschkow cells • Foci of T-lymphocytes • Necrosed collagen fibers
12th–16th week	Late fibrotic stage	• Fibrosis of Aschoff bodies occurs • Eventually, cellularity of Aschoff body decreases and it is replaced by a small fibrocollagenous scar

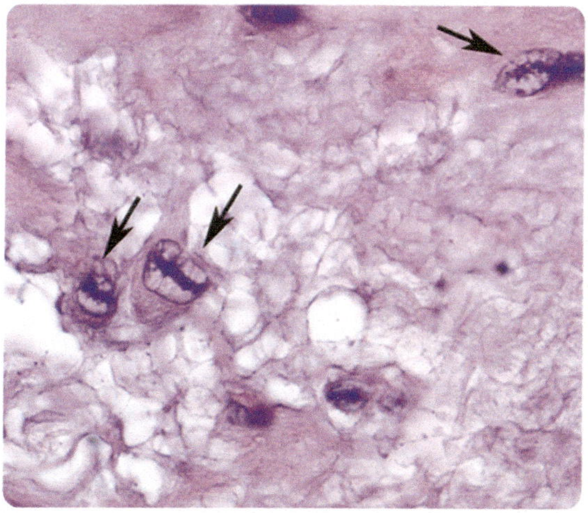

Fig. 1.6: Anitschkow cells/Caterpillar cells (arrows): Present in the center of Aschoff bodies and identified by the presence of linear condensation of nuclear chromatin. Image reprinted with permission from Allen Patrick Burke, MD, University of Maryland School of Medicine, published by Medscape Reference (emedicine.medscape.com; 2013, available at: emedicine.medscape.com/article/1962779-overview)

Which ventricle will be affected more?

- Long-standing congestive changes in the lungs induce pulmonary vascular and parenchymal changes, eventually leading to *right ventricular hypertrophy.*
- The left ventricle is largely unaffected by an isolated mitral stenosis.

Which are the clinical findings of cardiac involvement in RHD?

Inflammation of cardiac layers	*Clinical findings*
Pericarditis	Audible friction rub
Myocarditis	Unexplained CHF/ cardiomegaly; almost always associated with valvular involvement
Endocarditis/valvulitis	Presence of murmur of mitral regurgitation

Which is the most common ECG change found in RHD?

First degree AV block.

How will you diagnose RF and RHD?

2002–2003 WHO criteria for the diagnosis of rheumatic fever and rheumatic heart disease (based on the revised Jones criteria):

Diagnostic categories	*Criteria*
Primary episode of RF[a]	Two major * or one major and two minor **manifestation **plus** evidence of a preceding Group A streptococcal infection***
Recurrent attacks of RF in a patient **without** established rheumatic heart disease[b]	Two major or one major and two minor manifestation **plus** evidence of a preceding Group A streptococcal infection
Recurrent attacks of RF in a patient **with** established rheumatic heart disease	Two minor manifestation **plus** evidence of a preceding Group A streptococcal infection[c]
Rheumatic chorea Insidious onset rheumatic carditis	Other major manifestations of evidence of Group A streptococcal infection not required
Chronic valve lesions of RHD (patients presenting for the first time with pure mitral stenosis or mixed mitral valve disease and/or aortic valve disease)[d]	Do not require any other criteria to be diagnosed as having rheumatic heart disease
* Major manifestations	— Carditis — Polyarthritis — Chorea — Erythema marginatum — Subcutaneous nodules
** Minor manifestations	— Clinical: Fever, polyarthralgia — Laboratory: Elevated acute phase reactants (erythrocyte sedimentation rate or leukocyte count)
*** Supporting evidence of a preceding streptococcal infection within the last 45 days	— Electrocardiogram: Prolonged P-R interval — Elevated or rising antistreptolysin-O or other streptococcal antibody, or — A positive throat culture, or — Rapid antigen test for Group A streptococcus, or — Recent scarlet fever

[a] Patients may present with polyarthritis (or with only polyarthralgia or monoarthritis) and with several (3 or more) other minor manifestation, together with evidence of recent Group A streptococcal infection. Some of these cases may later turnout to be rheumatic fever. It is prudent to consider them as cases of 'probable rheumatic fever' (once other diagnoses are excluded and advise regular secondary prophylaxis. Such patients require close follow-up and regular examination of the heart. This cautious approach is particularly suitable for patients in vulnerable age groups.

[b] Infective endocarditis should be excluded.

[c] Some patients with recurrent attacks may not fulfill these criteria.

[d] Congenital heart disease should be excluded.

What are the effects of mitral stenosis on different organs?

Organs	Effects
Heart	
Left ventricle:	Normal
Right ventricle	
Left atrium	Dilation and hypertrophy
Right atrium	
Lungs	The lungs are heavy, voluminous, firm and **brownish** in color
Liver	**Nutmeg liver** (cut surface shows alternate dark and pale area, major cause is congestive cardiac failure)
Spleen	Congestive splenomegaly
Kidney	Congestion and proteinuria
Peritoneum	Ascites

What are the complications of mitral stenosis?

1. Recurrent hemoptysis
2. Congestive cardiac failure
3. Atrial fibrillation
4. Embolism
5. Dysphagia
6. Subacute bacterial endocarditis (Fig. 1.7).

Subacute bacterial endocarditis (SABE)

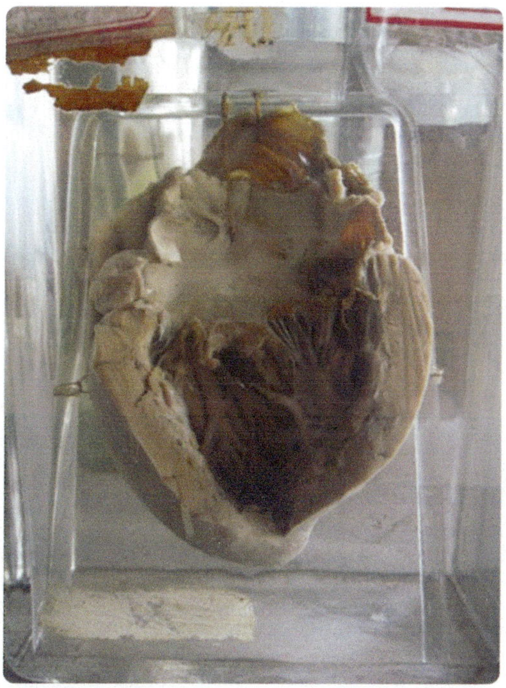

Fig. 1.7: Subacute bacterial endocarditis (SABE)

Description

This is a specimen of heart showing evidence of damage to valve cusps and having vegetations which are brownish in color.

- So the specimen is identified as "Subacute bacterial endocarditis" (Fig. 1.7).

What are the causative bacteria?

Subacute bacterial endocarditis is usually caused by low virulence organism. For example:

1. *Strep. viridans* (most common)
2. *Strep. faecalis*
3. HACEK group of bacteria (Haemophilus, Actinobacillus, Cardiobacterium, Eikenella, and Kingella).

What is the most common site of vegetation?

Damaged mitral valve after a previous episode of rheumatic heart disease (RHD) (Fig. 1.8).

What are the known conditions that expose the heart to an episode of SABE?

1. A previously damaged heart
2. Previous episode(s) of bacteremia.

What are the risk factors for SABE?

1. Mitral valve prolapse
2. Degenerative calcific valvular stenosis
3. Bicuspid aortic valve
4. Artificial (prosthetic) valves.

Describe the pathogenesis of SABE.

- Transient low virulence bacteremia has minimal ill effects on a normal endocardium.
- But when the bacteria get implanted on a previously damaged valve/mural endocardium, they produce vegetations.
- SABE is thought to be a *type 3 hypersensitivity reactio*n (i.e. antigen antibody complexes; when not cleared adequately by immune cells, gives rise to an inflammatory reaction).

What is the typical microscopic picture of a SABE?

- Microscopically, the vegetations of a

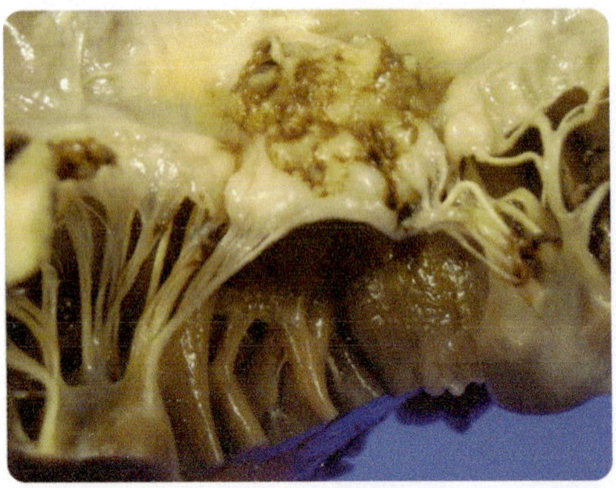

Fig. 1.8: Mitral valve: Endocarditis with large vegetation on the atrial aspect of the valve. The underlying chordae are relatively unremarkable. Image reprinted with permission from Allen Patrick Burke, MD, University of Maryland School of Medicine, published by Medscape Reference (emedicine.medscape.com; 2013, available at: emedicine.medscape.com/article/1954887-overview)

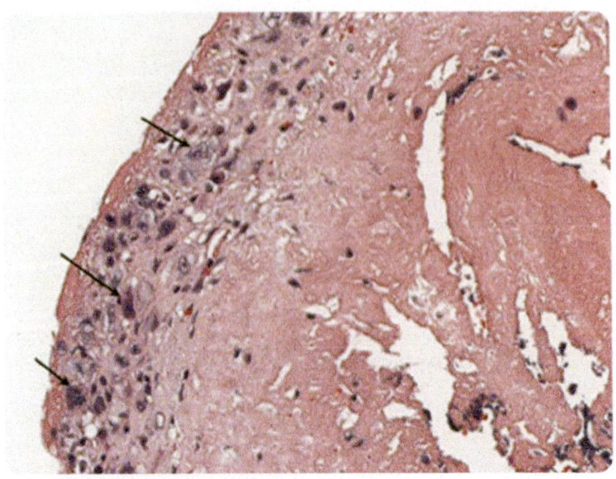

Fig. 1.9: Infective endocarditis, surface of valve leaflet with fibrin and macrophages (arrows), which are seen in the acute and subacute phases of inflammation. Image reprinted with permission from Allen Patrick Burke, MD, University of Maryland School of Medicine, published by Medscape Reference. (emedicine.medscape.com; 2013, available at: emedicine.medscape.com/article/1954887-overview)

typical SABE have granulation tissue indicative of healing at their bases.
- With time, fibrosis, calcification and a chronic inflammatory infiltrate (presence of macrophages) can develop (Fig. 1.9).

What are the complications of SABE?

Site	*Complications*
Cardiac	• Focal degenerative changes • Necrosis of the myocardium • Rupture of the interventricular septum
Extracardiac	• Microthromboemboli formation • Retinal hemorrhages (Roth spots) • Painful subcutaneous nodules on the pulp of the digits (Osler's node) • Painless erythematous lesions of palm/sole (Janeway lesions) • Hematuria due to immune complex • Glomerulonephritis

What are the differentiating points between SABE and acute bacterial endocarditis?

Acute bacterial endocarditis	*Subacute bacterial endocarditis*
It is caused by highly virulent organism (e.g. *Staph. aureus*)	It is caused by organism of low virulence (e.g *Strep. viridans*)
It affects the normal heart	It affects only the previously damaged heart valve/mural endocardium
It is associated with multiple pyogenic abscess formation as the emboli contains virulent organism	Here usually no/single abscess is seen
The microscopic picture is of an **acute inflammation** as the valve cusps show congestion/necrosis/ulceration/perforation	The microscopic picture is of a **chronic inflammation** as the vegetations show granulation tissue/fibrosis/calcification/a chronic inflammatory infiltrate

Atheroma

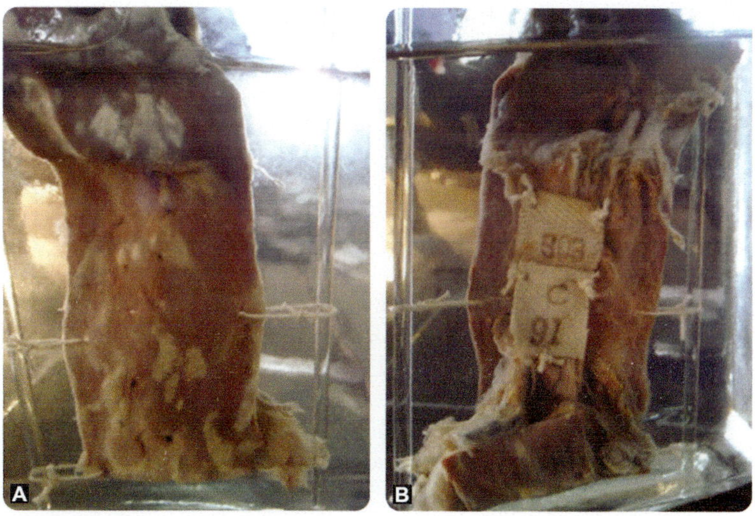

Figs 1.10A and B: Atheroma

Description

- Specimen showing a large artery cut open to expose intimal surface (identified by ostia of branch vessels).
- The intima is showing **raised pearly white plaque** close to the opening of ostia of branch vessels.
  - So, the specimen is identified as "**Atheroma of a large blood vessel**' (Figs 1.10A and B).

What are the arteries commonly affected?

1. Abdominal aorta
2. Coronary arteries
3. Cerebral arteries.

Name some of the common risk factors for atheroma formation.

1. Hyperlipidemia
2. Hypertension
3. Diabetes mellitus
4. Cigaret smoking.

Mention the main steps of "Response to injury" hypothesis of atherosclerosis.

According to this hypothesis, atherosclerosis is a chronic inflammatory response and also an attempt of healing of the arterial wall to endothelial injury. The steps are as follows: (Figs 1.11 and 1.12)

Name the different stages in the evolution of atheroma.

1. Fatty streaks
2. Atherosclerotic plaque
3. Complicated atherosclerotic plaques.

Describe the different stages in the evolution of atheroma.

Fatty streaks:

- Fatty streaks are the earliest lesions in the evolution of atherosclerosis.
- They are composed of LDL-filled foamy macrophages (or foam cells) located beneath the endothelium of an artery.
- At first, they are visualized as multiple minute flat yellow spots, but eventually they coalesce to form elongated streaks.
- These lesions do not cause any flow disturbance and are clinically silent.

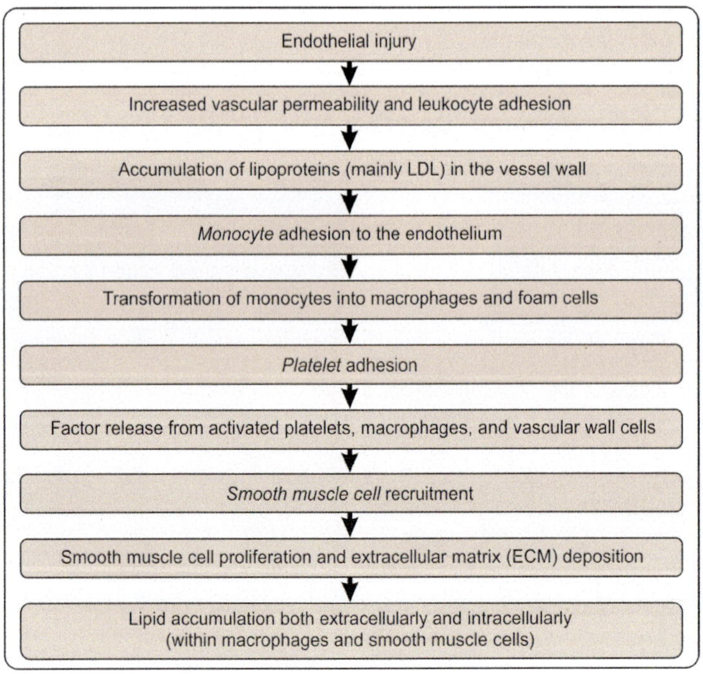

Fig. 1.11: Pathogenesis of atherosclerosis (steps)

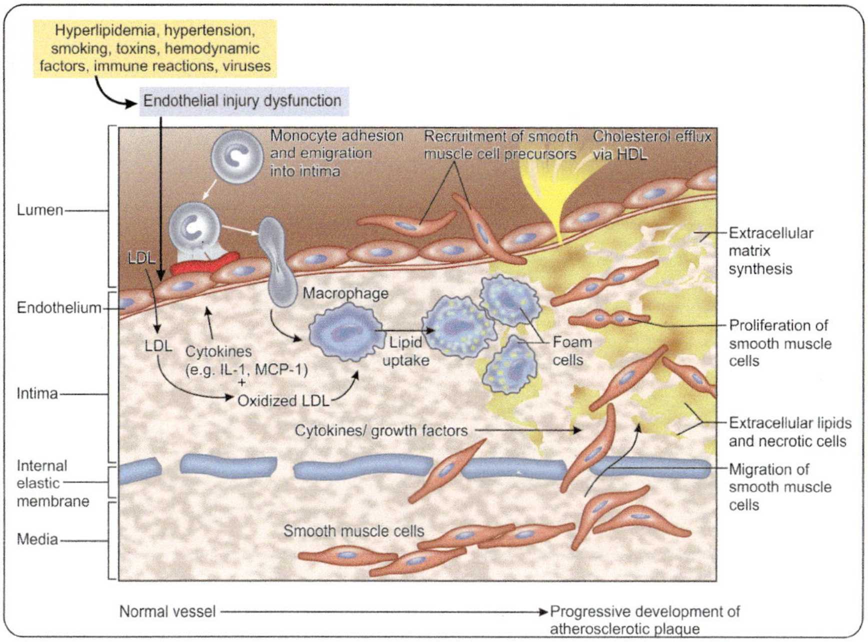

Fig. 1.12: Pathogenesis of atherosclerosis (graphical representation)

Atherosclerotic plaque:

- They are white to yellow plaques on the lumen of the artery; about 0.3–1.5 cm in diameter, resulting from lipid accumulation and intimal thickening.
- A typical atherosclerotic plaque consists of the following components (Fig. 1.13).

Components	Contents
A necrotic core at the center	• Cell debris • Cholesterol • Cholesterol esters • Foam cells
A fibrous cap in the periphery	• Collagen and elastin • Smooth muscle cells • Foam cells • Macrophages • Lymphocytes • New blood vessels

Complicated atherosclerotic plaque:

A mature atherosclerotic plaque is susceptible to the following complications:

1. Ulceration of the plaque.
2. Rupture of the plaque (an unstable plaque ruptures easily).
3. Thrombosis (due to plaque rupture and release of highly procoagulant substances*into the bloodstream).
4. Emboli formation (due to plaque rupture).
5. Hemorrhage into the plaque (due to presence of weak new vessels in the fibrous cap).
6. Aneurysm formation (due to ischemia of the media of the blood vessels and resulting weakness of the vessel wall).

The major consequences of a complicated atherosclerotic plaque are:

Involved.organs	Consequence
Heart	Myocardial infarction
Brain	Cerebral infarction
Lower extremity	Gangrene of the legs
Great vessels	Aneurysm of the aorta

(*Example: Tissue factor and plasminogen activator Inhibitor (PAI) from endothelial cells and release of active granules from platelets)

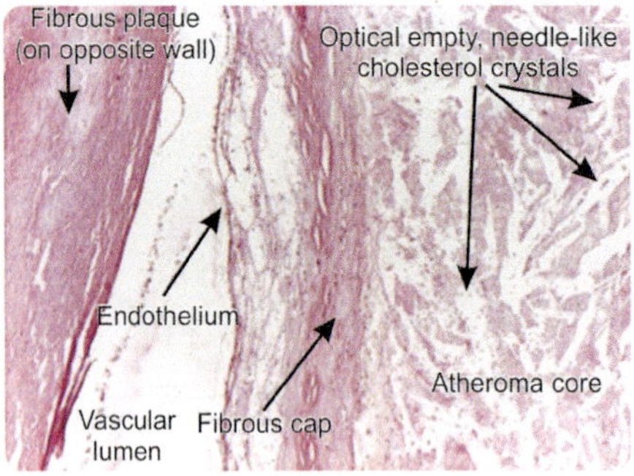

Fig. 1.13: Structure of an atherosclerotic plaque: Reproduced under the permission of Dr Mihai Danciu, Gr T Popa University of Medicine and Pharmacy, Iasi, Romania

What do you mean by a stable and an unstable plaque?

The atheromatous plaques may have two types of progression (Fig. 1.14):

Stable plaques:
- The atheromatous plaques may grow slowly due to gradual accumulation of lipids in the foam cells.
- The fibrous cap in these plaques gets matured and thickened, so they are not susceptible to rupture.
  – So they are called "Stable" plaques.

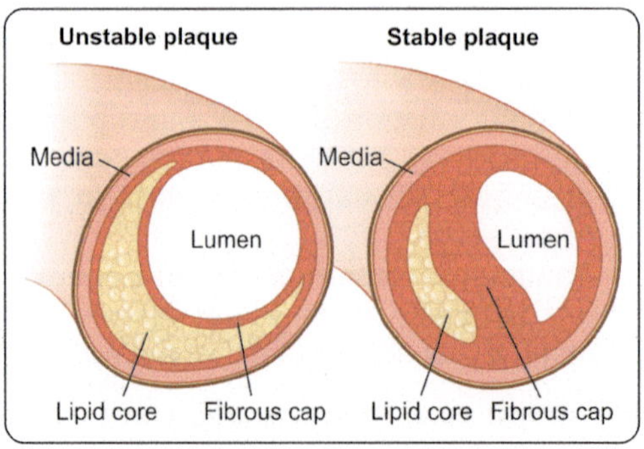

Fig. 1.14: Structure of a stable plaque and an unstable plaque vulnerable to complications like rupture, ulceration and hemorrhage

Unstable plaques:
- The atheromatous plaques may grow rapidly due to rapid accumulation of lipids in the foam cells.
- The fibrous cap in these plaques is thin and prone to early rupture.
  – So they are called "Unstable" plaques.

It should be remembered that once an atheromatous plaque gets ruptured, it rapidly activates platelets and the clotting cascades, rapidly resulting in an acute thrombotic event.

How does an atheroma narrow the blood vessels?

1. By presence of raised plaque
2. Thrombosis of the ulcerated plaque
3. Hemorrhage under the plaque pushing it up
4. Rupture of the plaque.

Left ventricular hypertrophy

Description

- This is a specimen of heart showing a transverse cut section of the left ventricle, which is highly thickened.
- The tendinous cords are also showing extensive thickening.
- The size of the left ventricle is increased.
- There is massive dilation of the left ventricle.
  – So, the specimen is identified as "Left ventricular hypertrophy" (Fig. 1.15).

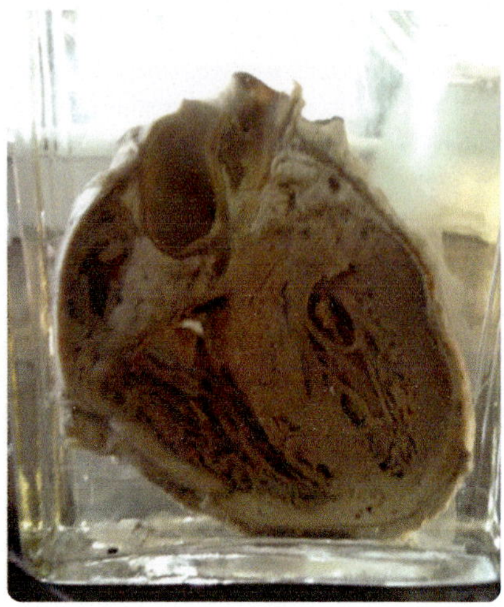

Fig. 1.15: Left ventricular hypertrophy

What is the main cause of left ventricular hypertrophy?

Left-sided heart failure, which is most often caused by:

1. Ischemic heart disease
2. Hypertension
3. Aortic and mitral valvular diseases.

What are the pathogenesis and consequences of cardiac hypertrophy?

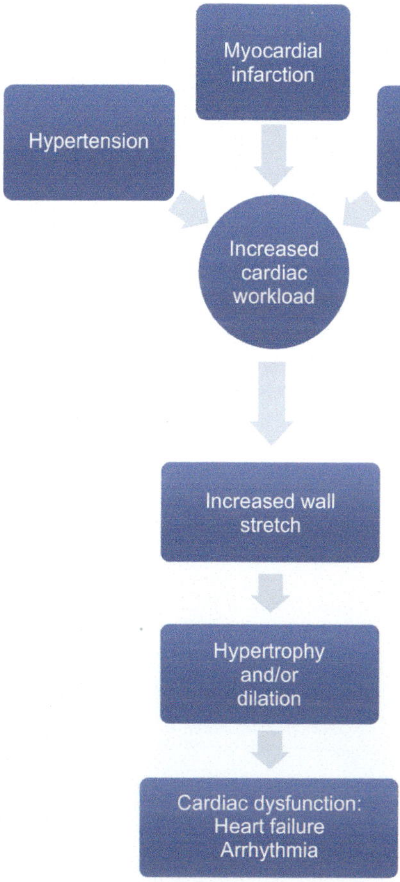

Fig. 1.16: Pathogenesis and consequences of cardiac hypertrophy

What are the changes seen in the lungs in a case of LVH?

1. Heavy and wet lungs:

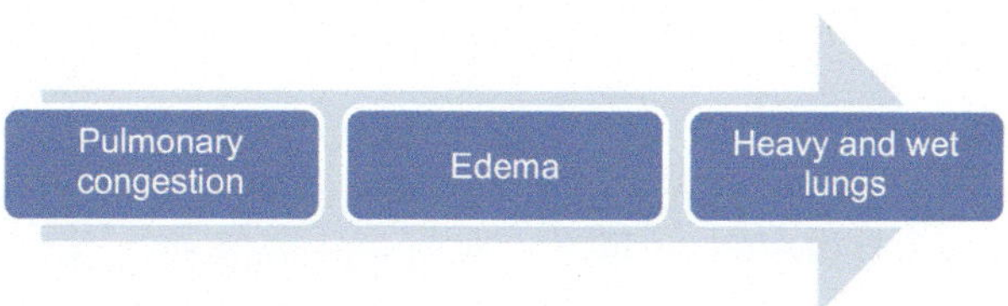

Fig. 1.17: Pulmonary congestion is characteristic of left-sided heart failure

2. Formation of "Heart failure cells":

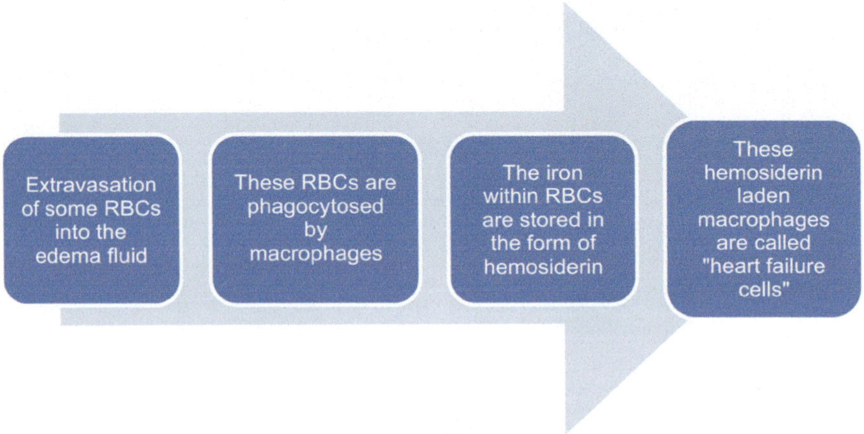

Fig. 1.18: Heart failure cells

3. The other definite changes are:

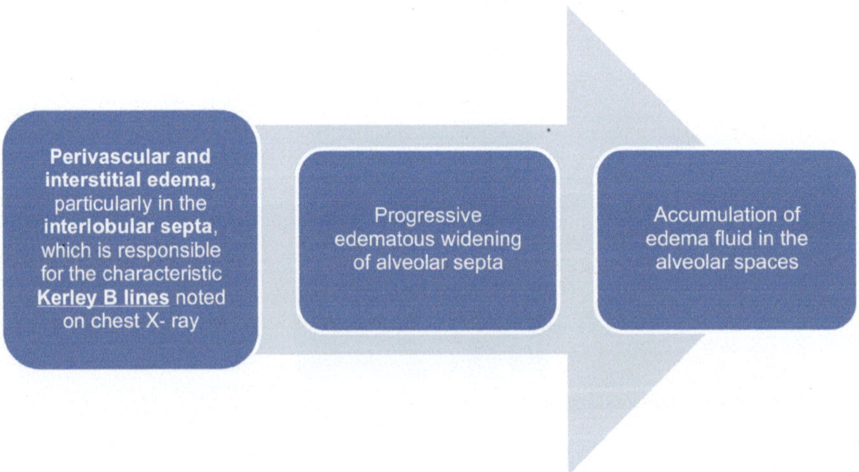

Fig. 1.19: Sequential events leading to pulmonary edema in left-sided heart failure

What are Kerley B lines?

They are 1–2 cm thin pulmonary opacities seen perpendicular to the pleural surface, representing thickened subpleural interlobular septa (Fig. 1.20).

Common causes:

1. Congestive cardiac failure
2. Pulmonary fibrosis
3. Recurrent pulmonary edema.

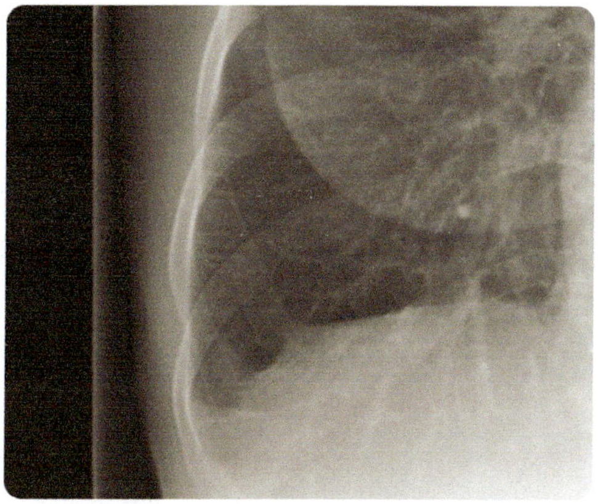

Fig. 1.20: Kerley B lines: Reproduced under the permission of Dr Sajoscha Sorrentino and Radiopaedia.org

What are the changes seen in other organs?

Organs	Changes
Kidney	Prerenal azotemia (because of the hypoperfusion of kidney, excretion of nitrogenous products increases significantly)
Brain	Hypoxic encephalopathy (due to cerebral hypoxia)

Fibrinous pericarditis

Description

- It is a specimen of heart showing the pericardium at its outer surface.
- The surface is dry.
- The surface is also showing a **fine granular roughening**.
  - So, the specimen is identified as "Fibrinous pericarditis" (Figs 1.21A and B).

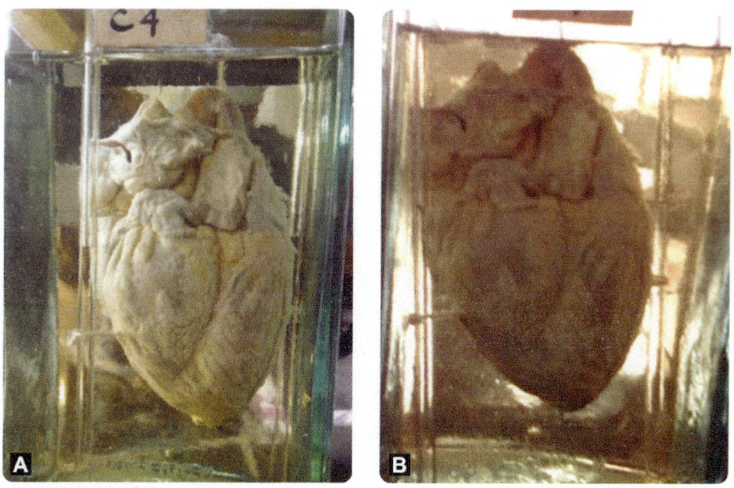

Figs 1.21A and B: Fibrinous pericarditis

What are the common causes of fibrinous pericarditis?

1. AMI
2. Postinfarction syndrome
3. Uremia
4. Chest radiation
5. Rheumatic fever
6. SLE
7. Trauma.

What is the most striking clinical sign of fibrinous pericarditis?

A loud pericardial friction rub.

How will you classify pericarditis?

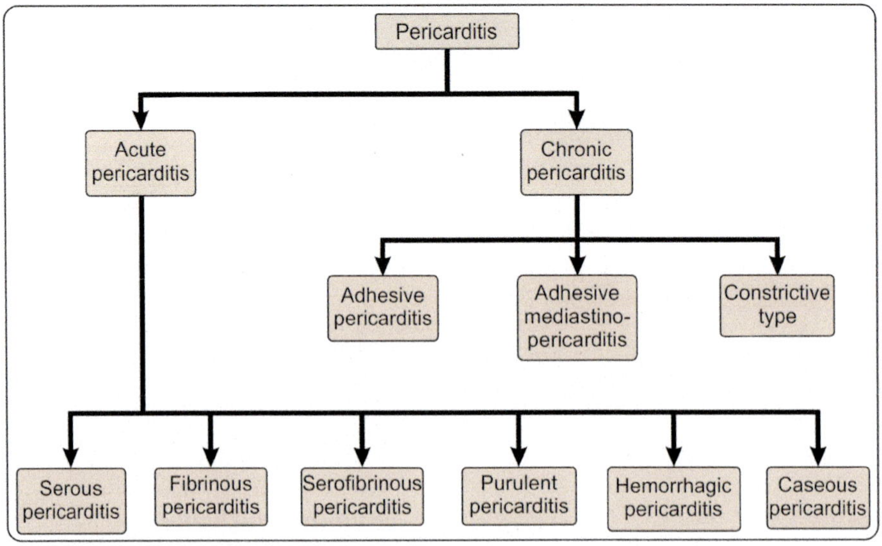

Fig. 1.22: Classification of pericarditis

Describe the differentiating features of different types of pericarditis.

Acute pericarditis

Types	*Etiology*	*Differentiating features*
Serous pericarditis	Characteristically of a sterile origin (SLE, rheumatic fever, tumors, uremia, viral infection, etc.)	Scant epicardial/pericardial mild inflammatory infiltrate
Fibrinous pericarditis	Most common type of pericarditis causes are described previously	Dry surface with a fine granular roughening
Serofibrinous pericarditis	Acute viral infection	Presence of large amount of yellow/ brown turbid exudate (filled with RBC, WBC, and fibrin)
Purulent pericarditis	Direct extension from adjacent infection sites (pneumonia/empyema/lung abscess, etc.). Most common agents are staphylococci, streptococci and pneumococci	Erythematous granular surface with extensive purulent exudate

Contd...

Contd...

Types	*Etiology*	*Differentiating features*
Hemorrhagic pericarditis	Most commonly seen after cardiac surgery; also associated with TB/ malignancy	Exudate is predominantly composed of blood admixed with fibrinous/purulent exudate
Caseous pericarditis	Caused by direct extension of tubercle bacilli from lymph nodes	Eventually leads to fibrocalcific constrictive pericarditis

Chronic pericarditis

Types	*Etiology*	*Differentiating features*
Adhesive pericarditis	Mostly seen in rheumatic heart disease (RHD)	Adhesion between parietal and visceral pericardium that does not impair cardiac function significantly
Adhesive mediastino-pericarditis	Seen after an episode of purulent pericarditis/cardiac surgery/ irradiation to the mediastinum	Adhesion between 2 layers of pericardium as well as between parietal pericardium and adjacent mediastinal structures; compelling the heart to contract against all the adhesive structures; eventually leading to hypertrophy and dilation
Constrictive pericarditis	Tuberculosis is the most common cause	There is marked thickening and scarring of parietal pericardium, causing the heart to lose its capacity to increase cardiac output in response to increased demand in the peripheral circulation

CHAPTER

2 Gastrointestinal Tract

Stomach

Before going into detail of description about the stomach specimens, we are briefly recapitulating the various parts of stomach, as it will help you to understand the site of involvement of diseases (Fig. 2.1).

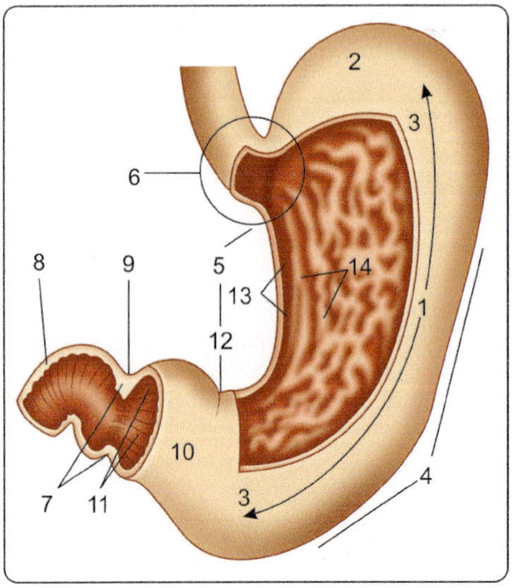

Fig. 2.1: 1. Body of stomach, 2. Fundus, 3. Anterior wall 4. Greater curvature, 5. Lesser curvature, 6. Cardia 7. Pyloric sphincter (valve), 8. Duodenum, 9. Pylorus, 10. Pyloric antrum, 11. Pyloric canal, 12. Angular notch, 13. Gastric canal, 14. Rugal folds

Peptic ulcer

Description

This is a specimen cut open along the greater curvature of stomach, showing mucosal ulcer with the following features:

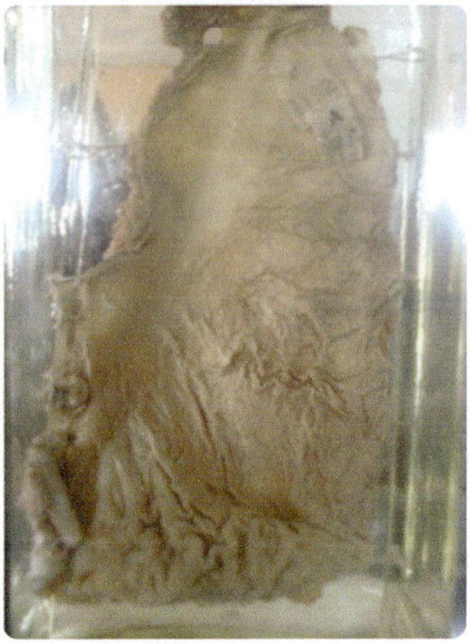

Fig. 2.2: Peptic ulcer

Features	Description
Location	Close to lesser curvature (95%)
Number	Usually single
Size	<2 cm in diameter
Shape	Oval/round
Margin	Sharply delineated
Edge	Thickened
Floor	Formed by serous/subserous layer and contains no muscle

– So, the above specimen is identified as "Peptic ulcer" (Fig. 2.2).

Why this is not a specimen of gastric carcinoma?

This is not a specimen of gastric carcinoma because in the ulcerative type of gastric carcinoma the following features are found:

Features	Description
Location	Greater curvature (most common)
Size	Usually >3 cm in diameter
Margin	Usually irregular
Edge	Thickened and everted
Floor	Formed by muscle layer

What are the sites where gastric ulcer may be found?

1. 1st part of duodenum (most common)
2. Stomach
3. Lower part of esophagus
4. Jejunum (after gastrojejunostomy)
5. Meckel's diverticulum (with gastric type of mucosa).

Describe the pathogenesis of peptic ulcer.

- Peptic ulcer is a complication of chronic gastritis.
- It is the result of a prolonged imbalance between the defensive and damaging forces of gastric mucosa and it arises when the damaging forces exceed the defensive ones.
- The pathogenesis of peptic ulcer is described below:

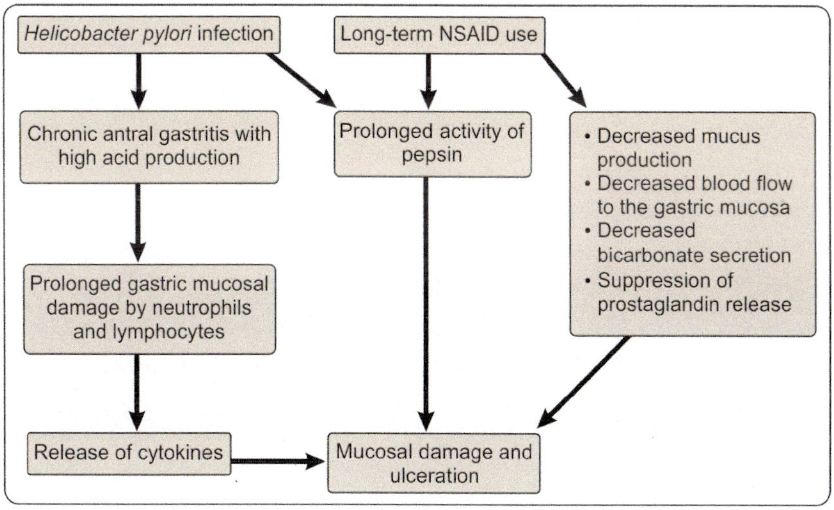

What are the main causes of duodenal ulcers?

- Duodenal ulcers are more frequent in individuals with:
  1. Alcoholic cirrhosis
  2. Chronic obstructive pulmonary disease (COPD)
  3. Chronic renal failure
  4. Hyperparathyroidism.
- In the last two conditions, *hypercalcemia stimulates gastrin production* and therefore increases acid secretion.

What will be the morphology of the above specimen?

- The classic peptic ulcer is characterized by a *round to oval, sharply punched-out defect.*
- The mucosal margin is usually level with the surrounding mucosa.
- *Hemorrhage* and *fibrin deposition* are seen frequently.
- The *base of peptic ulcers is smooth and clean as a result of peptic digestion of exudate.*
- *In active ulcers the base is formed by [above to downwards*: (Fig. 2.3)]

1. A predominantly neutrophilic inflammatory infiltrate
2. A thin layer of fibrinoid debris
3. Immature granulation tissue
4. Fibrous tissue.

- Exposed blood vessels may be seen in the ulcer base, typically within the scarred area. The vessel walls are thickened and thrombus may be seen.

What are the complications of peptic ulcer?

1. Perforation and peritonitis: It is a medical emergency.
2. Hemorrhage (leading to hematemesis and melena).
3. Penetration of ulcer into the adjacent structures.
4. Obstruction (due to scar formation) leading to pyloric stenosis.
5. Malignant transformation (very rare).

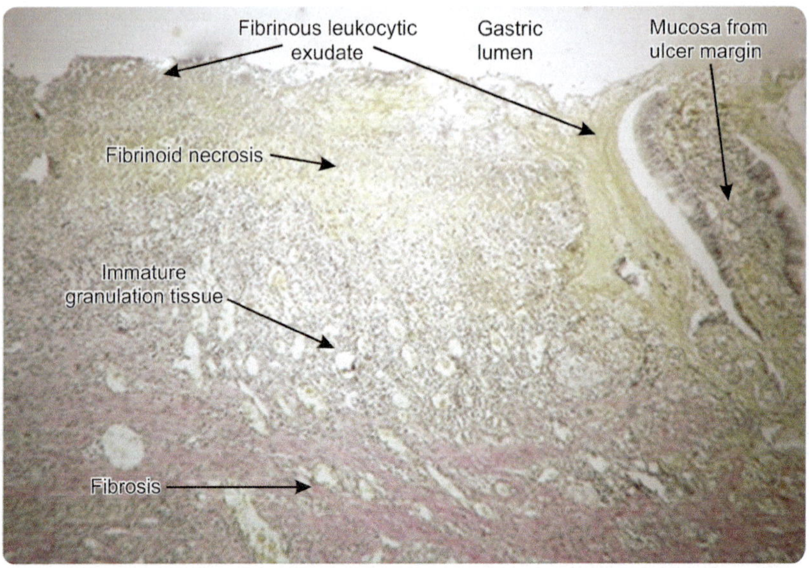

Fig. 2.3: Base of an active ulcer: Reproduced under the permission of Dr Mihai Danciu, Gr T Popa University of Medicine and Pharmacy, Iasi, Romania

What are the common clinical symptoms of peptic ulcer?

Usually the patients of peptic ulcer come to attention for the following clinical symptoms:

- Epigastric pain: Burning/continuous dull pain; often periodic
- Vomiting
- Bleeding
- Perforation and peritonitis (if complicated).

How can you diagnose peptic ulcer?

1. An upper GI endoscopy (preferably a gastroduodenoscopy) is considered to be the most accurate diagnostic test for peptic ulcer disease and considered to be the "Gold standard" for this purpose.
2. A urea breadth test: It is based on the demonstration of ammonia produced by *H.pylori* from urea by the enzyme "Urease".
3. A barium X-ray to detect any abnormality in the upper GIT (ulcer/ tumor/ hernia/ pouch/ stricture/ swallowing difficulty, etc.).
4. An ELISA test to detect antibodies against *H.pylori* in blood (has the disadvantage of getting a high numbers of false-positive reactions).

Can you name some drugs to treat peptic ulcer?

Two most effective triple drug regimens approved by FDA are:

1. Clarithromycin + Amoxicillin + Lansoprazole/Omeprazole (proton pump inhibitors).
2. Bismuth subsalicylate + Metronidazole + Tetracycline (BMT).

What is the relation between blood group and peptic ulcer?

Peptic ulcer is common among Group O persons.

Gastric carcinoma

Description

This is a specimen of stomach showing the following features (As shown in the following table) and the above specimen is identified as 'Gastric carcinoma' (Fig. 2.4).

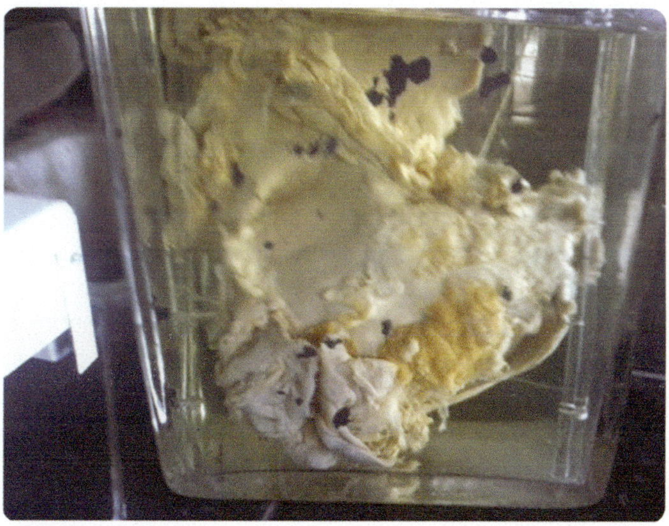

Fig. 2.4: Gastric carcinoma

Types	Description of the growth
Ulcerative type	Present on pylorus. Usually >3 cm in diameter, with thick and everted edge and hard indurated base formed by muscle
Fungating type	Large, cauliflower-like growth projecting in the lumen from mucosa, may cause pyloric obstruction when present in pylorus
Infiltrating type (leather bottle stomach)	Whole stomach is affected, length and cavity are grossly reduced, prominent mucosal fold and thickened wall

What are the types of gastric carcinoma?

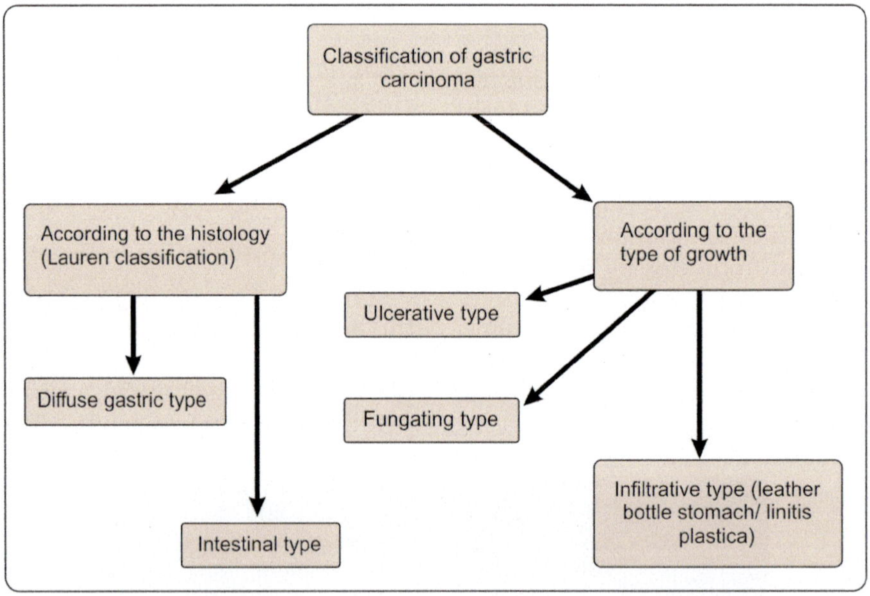

What is the pathogenesis of gastric carcinoma?

Pathogenesis of gastric carcinoma: Diffuse gastric type:

- E-cadherin is a protein that contributes to epithelial intercellular adhesion.
- Mutation in CDH1 gene (which codes E-cadherin) and subsequent loss of E-cadherin function seems to be a key step in the pathogenesis of diffuse gastric cancer.

Pathogenesis of gastric carcinoma: Intestinal type:

- Mutations/ microsatellite instability/ hypermethylation of various genes have been described in sporadic intestinal type gastric cancer:
  1. β-catenin
  2. TGFRII
  3. BAX
  4. IGFRII
  5. p16/INK4a.

What will be the morphology of the above specimen?

Types of gastric CA	*Diffuse gastric type*	*Intestinal type*
Features		
Gross morphology	Diffuse infiltrative growth pattern	Bulky tumors, they typically grow along broad cohesive fronts to form an exophytic mass/an ulcerated tumor
Histology	They are generally composed of discohesive cells that do not form glands but instead have large mucin vacuoles that push the nucleus to the periphery, creating a *signet-ring cell morphology* (Fig. 2.5A)	They usually show a *glandular morphology*; often associated with intestinal metaplasia of the surrounding area (Fig. 2.5B)

It should be remembered at the very beginning that most of the gastric carcinomas involve the gastric antrum and that the lesser curvature is involved more often than the greater curvature.

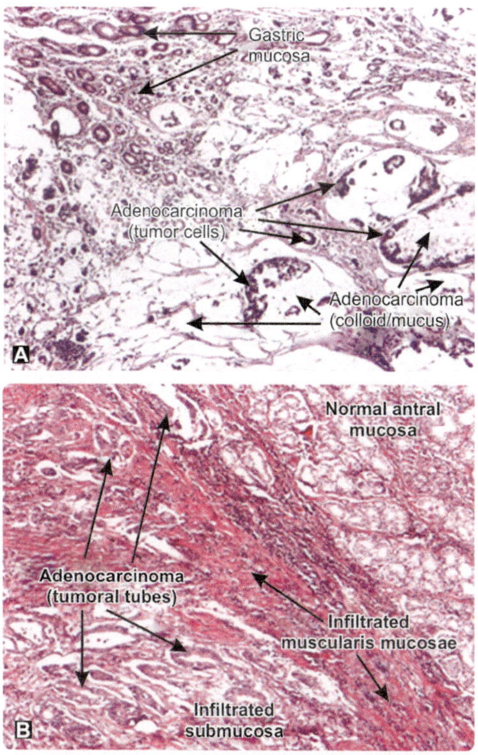

Figs 2.5 A and B: A. Morphology of diffuse type of gastric carcinoma: Presence of large amount of mucus and signet-ring cell morphology. B. Morphology of intestinal type of gastric carcinoma: Glandular morphology and intestinal metaplasia. Reproduced under the permission of Dr.Mihai Danciu, Gr T Popa University of Medicine and Pharmacy, Iasi, Romania

What is linitis plastica/ leather bottle stomach/ Brinton's disease/ diffuse stomach cancer?

It is a special type of stomach cancer characterized by involvement of the whole stomach, with a rigid and thickened wall caused by diffuse infiltration of the whole stomach by tumor cells and extensive fibrosis (Fig. 2.6).

Histologically, diffuse stomach cancer is characterized by a signet-ring cell morphology, caused by large mucin vacuoles pushing the nucleus to the periphery.

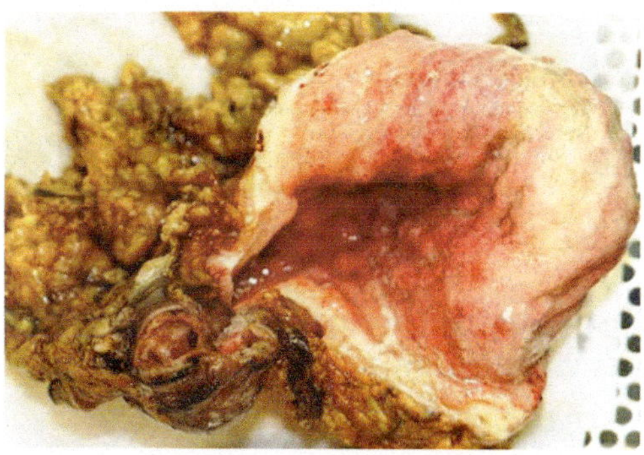

Fig. 2.6: Linitis plastica: Stomach opened longitudinally along the lesser curvature showing marked thickening of the gastric wall with mucosal congestion and decrease in rugal folds. Reproduced under the permission of Dr Andrew Ryan, MBBS, FRCPA

Which other cancers may create a linitis plastica appearance?

Breast and lung cancers that metastasize to the stomach may also create a linitis plastica-like appearance.

How hypochlorhydria helps in carcinogenesis?

- In presence of hypochlorhydria, the growth of *H.pylori* in stomach is promoted.
- This organism reduces dietary nitrate to nitrite.
- Then they convert the dietary amines to N-nitroso compounds (in the presence of nitrites).
- These N-nitroso compounds are highly carcinogenic and they are thought to be an important link between *H.pylori* and gastric cancer.

How can you differentiate between them?

Points	Ulcer cancer	Cancer ulcer
Definition	It is malignant transformation of a pre-existing chronic peptic ulcer	It is ulceration of a previously existed carcinoma
Finding of an endoscopic biopsy from the corner along with the base of ulcer	Only 1 or 2 bits will show the evidence of carcinoma	All the bits will show the evidence of carcinoma

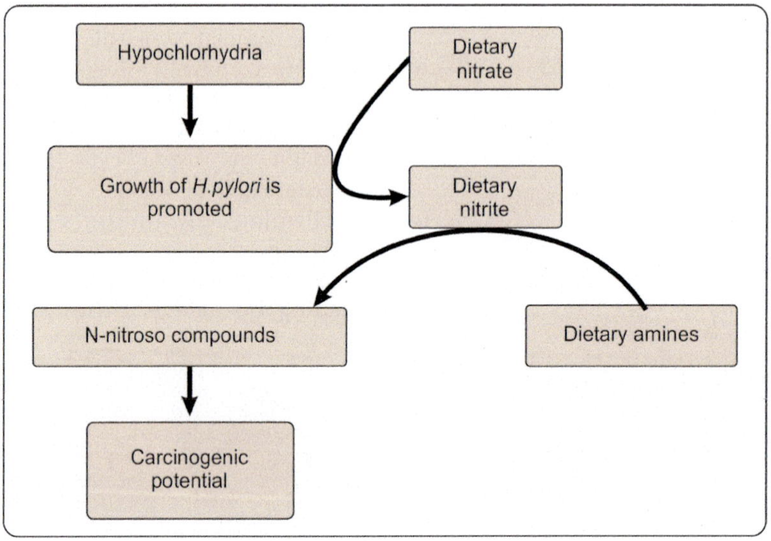

Name some common risk factors for gastric carcinoma.

1. Hypochlorhydria
2. *H.pylori* infection
3. Intestinal metaplasia.

What is the difference between ulcer cancer and cancer ulcer?

What are the modes of spread of gastric carcinoma?

1. Local spread.
2. Metastasis to the supraclavicular lymph node (also called Virchow's node).
3. Metastasis to periumbilical region to form a subcutaneous nodule, termed as Sister Mary Joseph nodule.

4. Hematogenous spread to liver and lung.
5. Transcelomic spread to ovaries producing Krukenberg's tumor.

Small intestine

Tuberculous ulcer

Description

It is a specimen showing ulcer of the small intestine with:

Features	Description
Long axis	Transversely disposed
Edge	Ragged and irregular
Floor	Showing small protuberances with no congestion of surrounding tissue
Serous coat	Showing presence of tubercles

- So, the above specimen is identified as "Tuberculous ulcer of the small intestine" (Fig. 2.7).

What is the etiological origin of intestinal tuberculosis?

Intestinal TB is usually a form of secondary TB.

What are the various pathogenetic mechanisms of intestinal TB?

- Swallowing of infected sputum
- Dissemination of primary pulmonary tuberculosis
- Ingestion of nonpasteurized milk (contaminated with bovine tuberculosis).

Why TB ulcer is most common in terminal ileum and cecum?

1. TB ulcer occurs in the areas of Peyer's patches and lymphoid follicles. Both terminal ileum and cecum are very rich in both.
2. Movement of gut is sluggish in these parts, so bacteria gets more time to settle down here.

What are the different morphological types of tuberculous lesions found in the gut?

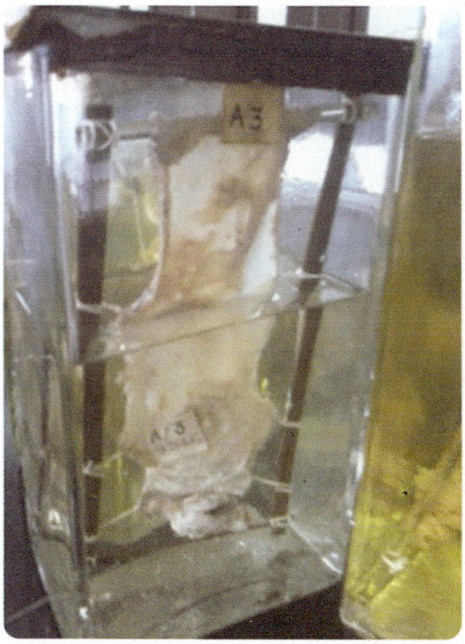

Fig. 2.7: Tuberculous ulcer

There are mainly 2 morphological types of intestinal TB:

A. Ulcerative type
B. Ulcerohypertrophic type.

It should be mentioned that there are no sharp differences between ulcerative and ulcerohypertrophic lesions and the two can occur at the same time.

Types of the lesion	*Features*
Ulcerative type (60%)	• Diseased areas are moderately indurated • Mesenteric fat is increased and mesenteric lymph nodes are enlarged • The circumference of the ulcer is studded with nodules of variable size • Characteristically, the established lesion consists of an *annular ulcer involving the entire circumference of a segment* and generally < 3 cm in length • The lumen in the affected region is markedly narrowed, often resulting in a stricture
Ulcerohypertrophic type (30%)	• Ulcerohypertrophic lesions usually affect the ileocecal region, the patient presenting with a large lump in the right iliac fossa • The ileocecal angle is distorted and often obtuse • *On opening, the wall is seen to be markedly thickened* (because of hypertrophy) • Mucosal changes are: a. Cobblestoning b. Pseudopolyposis c. Flattening of mucosal folds

What are the common complications of a TB ulcer?

1. Acute or chronic obstruction from stricture, adhesions or both is the most common complication.
2. Perforation with peritonitis, usually in the ileum proximal to a stricture.
3. Fistulae between loops of bowel/ between the bowel and the skin/ between adjacent organs.
4. Malabsorption from lymphatic obstruction.

What are the clinical presentations of intestinal TB?

- Abdominal pain and distension
- Fever
- Diarrhea
- Weight loss
- Obstruction
- Melena (bleeding from upper GI tract)
- A palpable mass in the abdomen
- Anorexia
- Night sweats.

Why TB ulcers are uncommon nowadays?

The incidence of primary intestinal TB has become very rare nowadays primarily due to control of bovine TB by pasteurization of milk.

Typhoid ulcer

Description

- This is a specimen of small intestine wall.
- Centrally there is a well-circumscribed raised ovoid lesion in longitudinal alignment, interpreted as an ulcerated Peyer's patch (unlike in tuberculous ulceration, in which the ulcers are arranged with their long axes transverse to the length of the bowel).
- A similar small rounded lesion is present at the lower-end of the specimen and still smaller nodules are scattered throughout.

Features	Description
Long axis	Oriented parallel to the long axis of the gut (longitudinally)
Shape	Oval
Edge	Regular, edematous, congested and raised
Floor	Pitted
Serous coat	Congested and having no tubercle

- So, the specimen is identified as "Typhoid ulcer" (Figs 2.8 and 2.9).

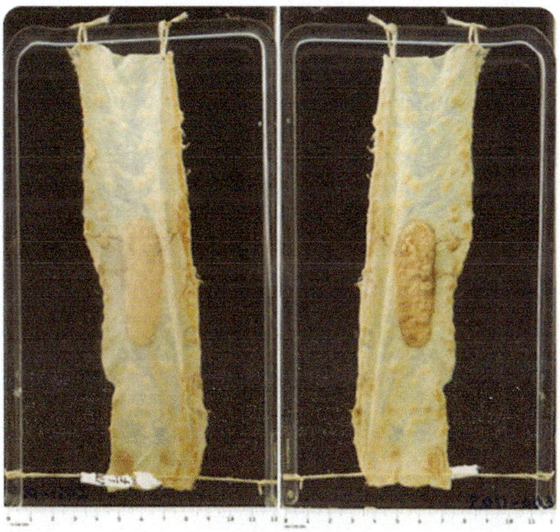

Fig. 2.8: Typhoid ulcer of small intestine. Reproduced under the permission of Department of Clinical Laboratory Sciences, University of Cape Town, South Africa

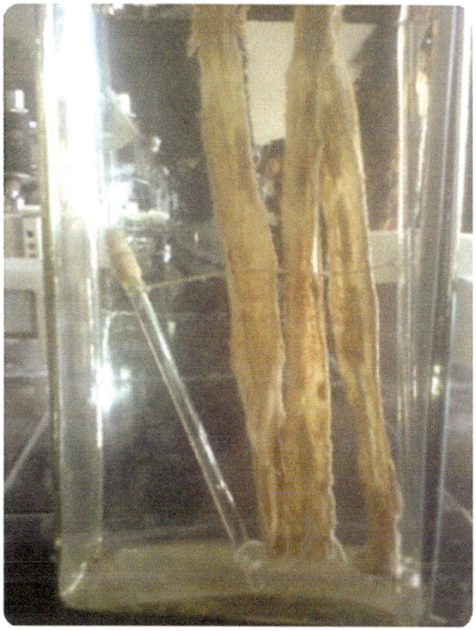

Fig. 2.9: Typhoid ulcer

What are the different phases of evolution of typhoid ulcer?

Phases	Features
Phase 1	*Hyperplasia* of lymphoid follicles
Phase 2	*Necrosis* of lymphoid follicles during the 2nd week involving both mucosa and submucosa
Phase 3	*Ulceration* in the long axis of the bowel with the possibility of perforation and hemorrhage
Phase 4	*Healing* takes place from the 4th week onward, and unlike tuberculosis of the bowel with its encircling ulcers, does not produce strictures

Describe the pathogenesis of typhoid ulcer.

- After being ingested, the organism *Salmonella typhi* reaches the small intestine, penetrates the mucosa and carried to the Peyer's patches of the lower small intestine.

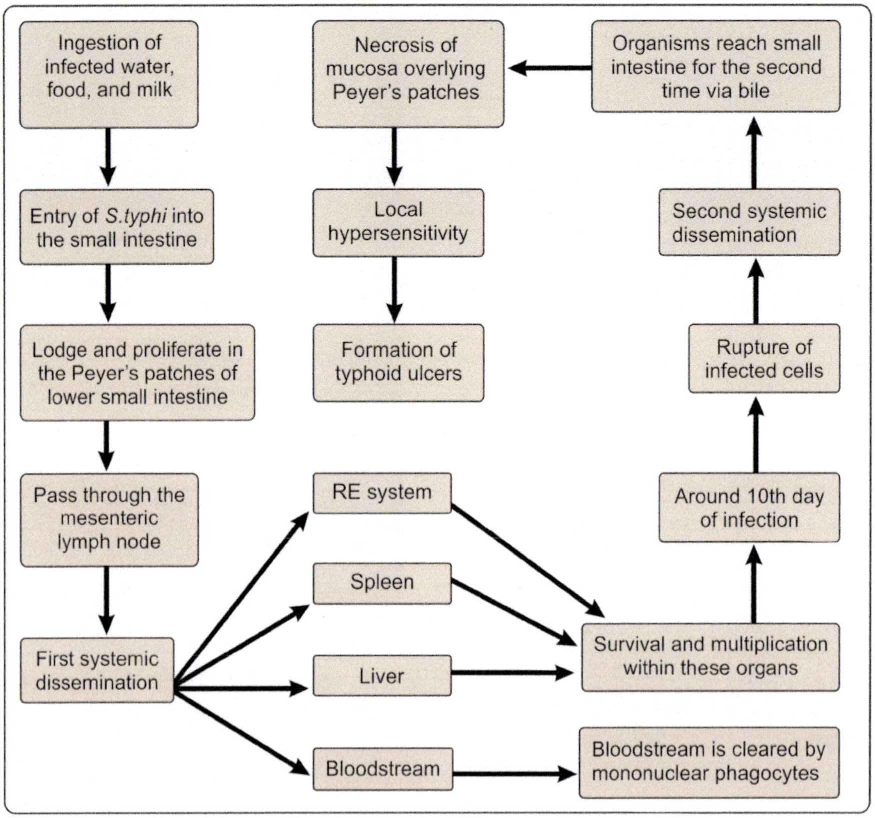

- Here they proliferate because of their special intracellular survival capability within the phagocytes and after passing through the mesenteric lymph nodes, they finally flood the bloodstream causing a systemic dissemination to the liver, spleen, and reticuloendothelial system.
- The bloodstream is immediately cleared by mononuclear phagocytes, but by the special capability of the organism mentioned above, they survive within these organs.
- By about 10th day of infection (varying from 1–3 weeks), the infected cells rupture and the bloodstream is flooded with large number of bacteria. This is the end of incubation period and the patient becomes seriously ill with septicemia.
- As the organisms reach the small intestine second time through bile, local hypersensitivity leads to necrosis of mucosa overlying Peyer's patches and results in formation of ulcer.

What is the most important histologic feature of a typhoid ulcer?

Presence of large number of macrophages, instead of neutrophils.

What is the most dangerous complication of a typhoid ulcer?

- In the 2nd or 3rd week of the illness, if the patient presents with severe generalized abdominal pain, it indicates a perforated typhoid ulcer.
- The patient will show classical features of peritonitis. (Abdominal pain, distension, fever, nausea, vomiting, loss of

appetite, diarrhea, thirst, low urine output, and constipation).

- So, any patient being treated for typhoid fever who shows a sudden deterioration accompanied by abdominal signs should be considered to have a typhoid perforation until proven otherwise.

What are the different lesions found in complicated typhoid fever?

Organs	Lesion
Intestine	Typhoid ulcer
Gallbladder	Cholecystitis
Liver	Typhoid nodules: Small, randomly scattered foci of parenchymal necrosis in which hepatocytes are replaced by macrophage aggregates
Spleen	Congestion and splenomegaly
Bones	Osteomyelitis
Skin	Typhoid rash
Respiratory system	Bronchitis and bronchopneumonia
Bone marrow	Suppression of leukopoiesis
Heart	Toxic myocarditis
CNS	Meningitis

Large intestine

Colon carcinoma

Description

It is a specimen of proximal colon showing polypoid, exophytic masses that extend along one wall of the large-caliber cecum and ascending colon.

- So, this specimen is identified as colon carcinoma (Fig. 2.10).

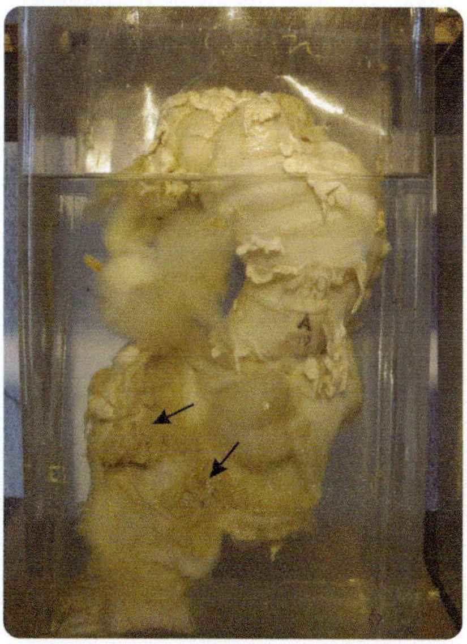

Fig. 2.10: Carcinoma of colon. Specimen of a part of colon: Lower part of it is cut open to show a projecting fungating polyploid growth (arrows) with glistening surface

What is the pathogenesis of colon cancer?

The pathogenesis of colon carcinoma has 2 pathways:

A. The classical adenoma-carcinoma sequence pathway (Fig. 2.11)
B. The microsatellite instability pathway (Fig. 2.12).
   - Both are being discussed briefly here in diagrams.

What is the morphology of colon carcinoma?

1. The tumors are composed of tall columnar cells.
2. The invasive component of these tumors elicits a strong stromal desmoplastic reaction, which is responsible for the characteristic firm consistency of the tumor.
3. Glandular morphology with abundant mucin production is associated with poor prognosis.

What are the most common sites of metastasis?

- As a result of portal drainage of the colon, liver is the most common site of metastatic lesions.
- But metastases may also involve the following structures:
  1. Regional lymph nodes
  2. Lungs
  3. Bones.

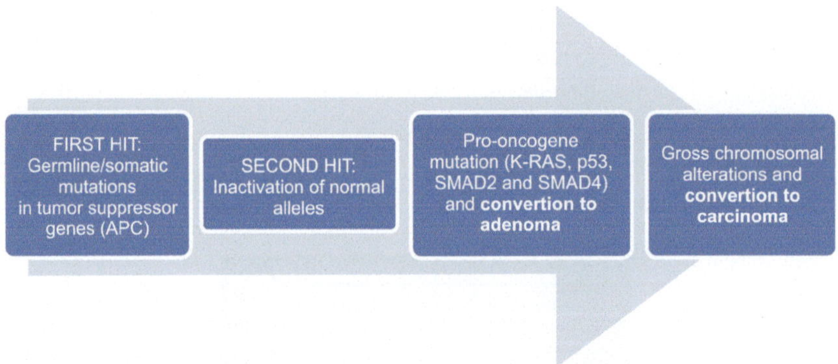

Fig. 2.11: The adenoma-carcinoma pathway

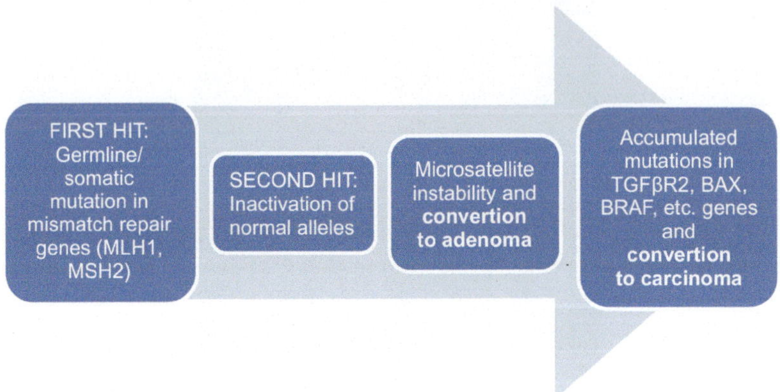

Fig. 2.12: The microsatellite instability pathway

What are the most common presenting features of colon carcinoma?

Colon cancers	Presenting features
Right-sided	Fatigue and weakness due to iron deficiency anemia
Left-sided	• Occult bleeding • Changes in bowel habits • Cramping left lower quadrant discomfort

Is "Beta catenin" gene mutated in colon cancer?

- The "Beta catenin" commonly mentioned in CA colon is actually the Beta catenin protein, not the Beta catenin gene.
- Mutations in the APC gene in CA colon (the adenoma carcinoma sequence pathway) causes accumulation of Beta catenin protein within the cell cytoplasm, which leads to persistent activation of a transcription factor named TCF within the nucleus. Beta catenin gene is never mutated in colon cancer.
- This causes abnormal cell proliferation and eventually leads to tumor formation.

In which cancers, the Beta catenin gene is actually mutated?

Mutations in Beta catenin gene are commonly associated with:

a. Hepatoblastoma
b. Hepatocellular carcinoma.

Name some of the genes which are mutated in colon cancer.

Types of colon cancer	Genes which are mutated
Hereditary colon cancer	• APC • Mismatch repair genes
Sporadic colon cancer	• MYC • K-RAS • SRC • erbB2 • P^{53} • APC • Mismatch repair genes

CHAPTER 3

Liver

Basic histological anatomy of liver

It should be mentioned that the histopathology of liver is usually discussed on the basis of a lobular architecture. So, in the schematic diagram drawn below (Fig. 3.1):

a. A lobule is oriented around the terminal hepatic vein (tributaries of hepatic vein).
b. The area in the vicinity of terminal hepatic vein is called "Centrilobular" area (Fig. 3.2B).
c. The area in the vicinity of portal tract is called "Periportal" area (Fig. 3.2A).

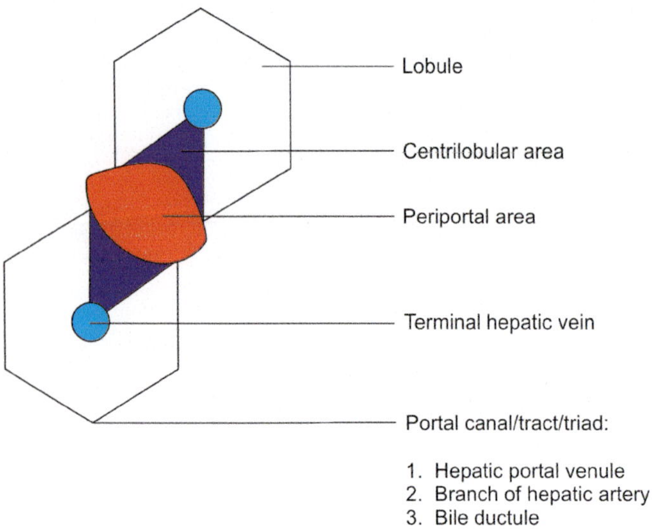

Fig. 3.1: Basic histopathological anatomy of liver

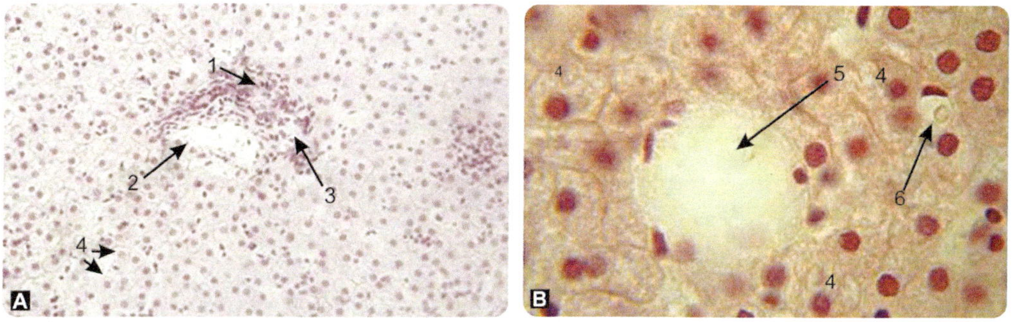

Figs 3.2A and B: Histological slides of liver stained with hematoxylin and eosin (H and E) showing A. Structure of a portal triad (1–Hepatic artery, 2–Portal vein, 3–Bile duct, 4–Hepatocytes) and B. Centrilobular area (4–Hepatocytes, 5–Terminal hepatic venule, 6–Hepatic sinusoid). Reproduced under the permission of Dr Andrei Gunin, Dept. of Histology, Chuvash State University, Rassia

Fatty liver

Description

It is a specimen of liver tissue showing:

Features	Description
Color	Pale yellow
Surface	Smooth
Capsule	Stretched
Margin	Rounded
Cut surface	Greasy (if fresh)
Consistency	Soft (if palpated)

- So, the above specimen is identified as "Fatty liver" (Figs 3.3A and B).

What do you mean by "Fatty liver"?

Fatty liver is a reversible condition where large vacuoles of triglyceride (TAG) accumulate within the hepatocytes.

What do you mean by "Steatosis"?

"Steatosis" is defined as abnormal retention of fat within a cell.

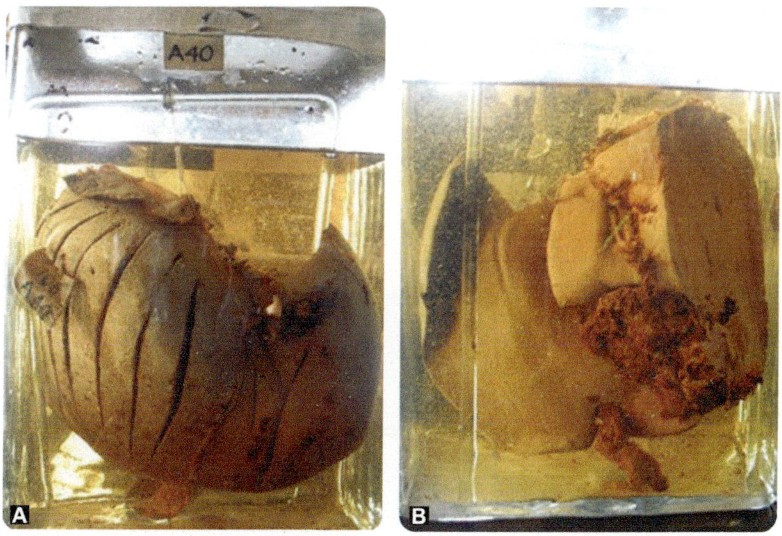

Figs 3.3A and B: Fatty liver. A. Front view and B. Back view

How can you classify fatty liver?

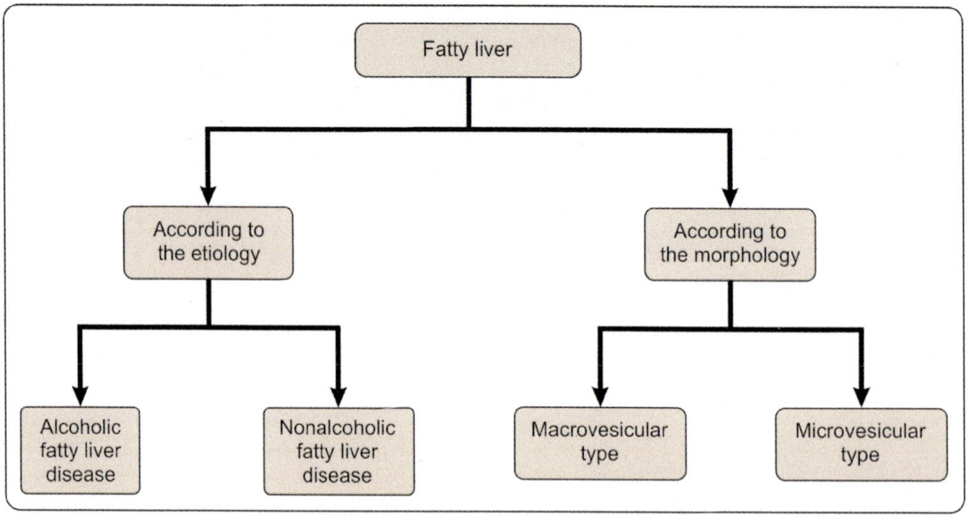

Describe the pathogenesis of alcoholic fatty liver disease/alcoholic steatosis.

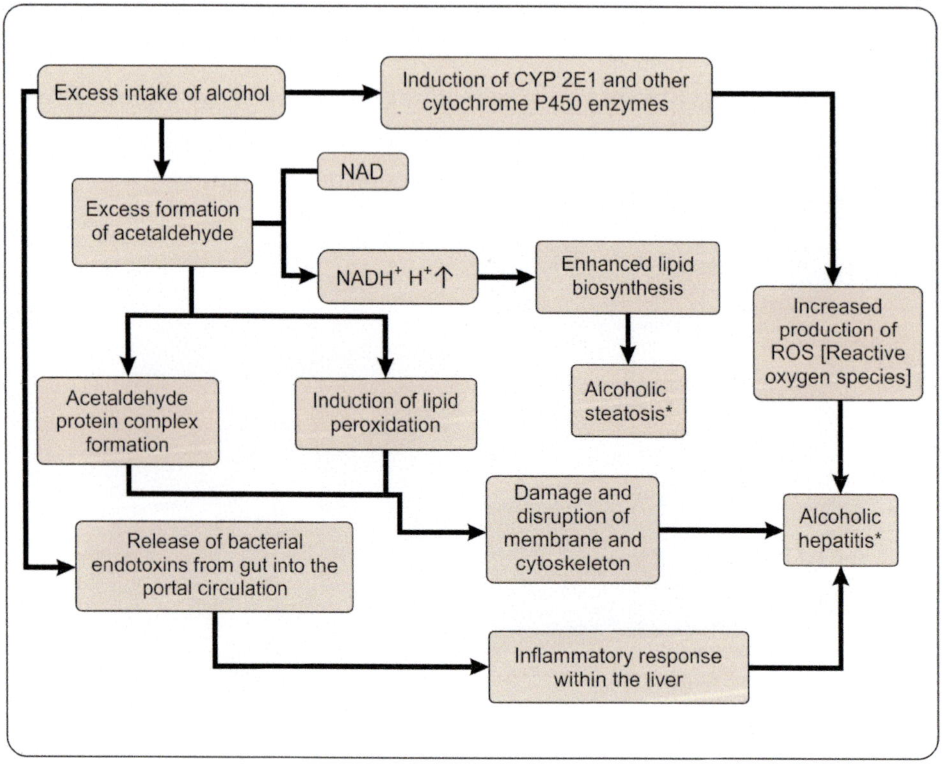

(*These 2 processes are together termed as "Alcoholic steatohepatitis").

What are the different pathologic stages in the progression of alcoholic steatohepatitis?

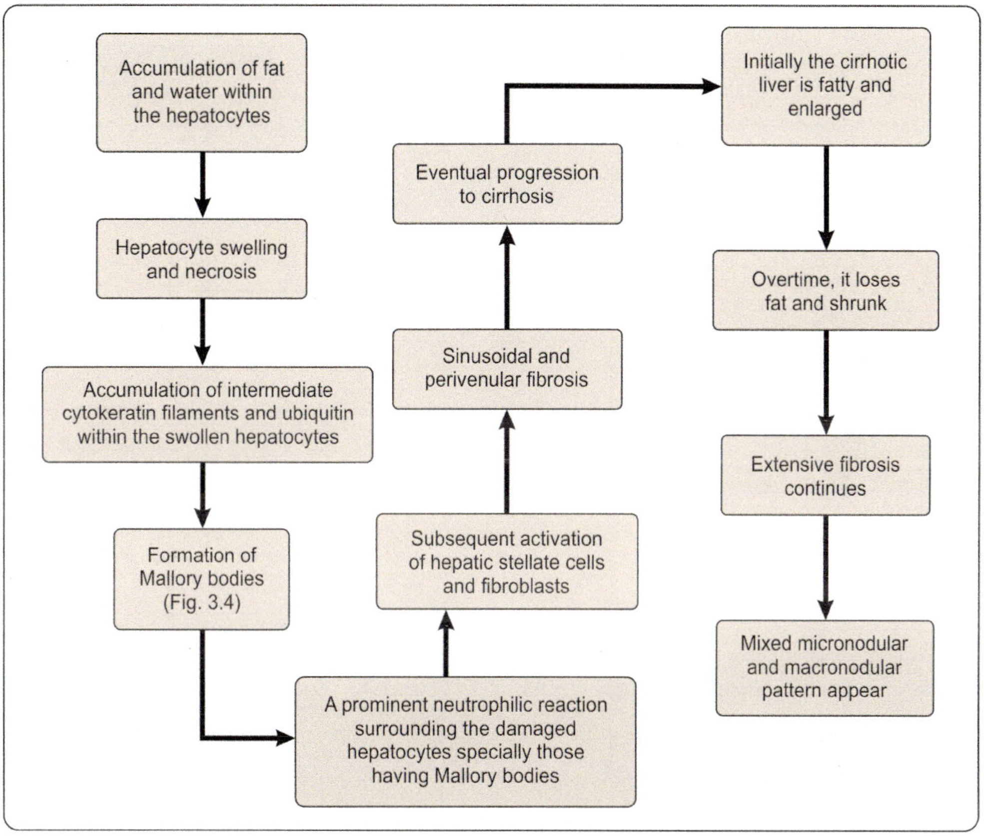

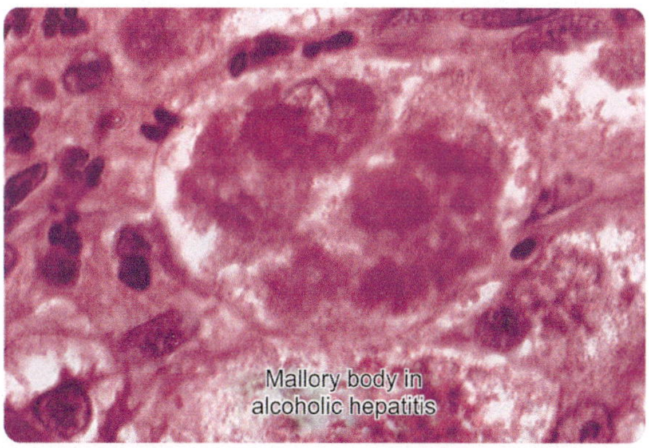

Fig. 3.4: Micrograph showing a Mallory body at the center of the image within a swollen hepatocyte. As they are highly eosinophilic in nature, they appear pink in H and E stain.(Reproduced under the permission of Joel Greenson, University of Michigan)

Describe the pathogenesis of nonalcoholic fatty liver disease (NAFLD).

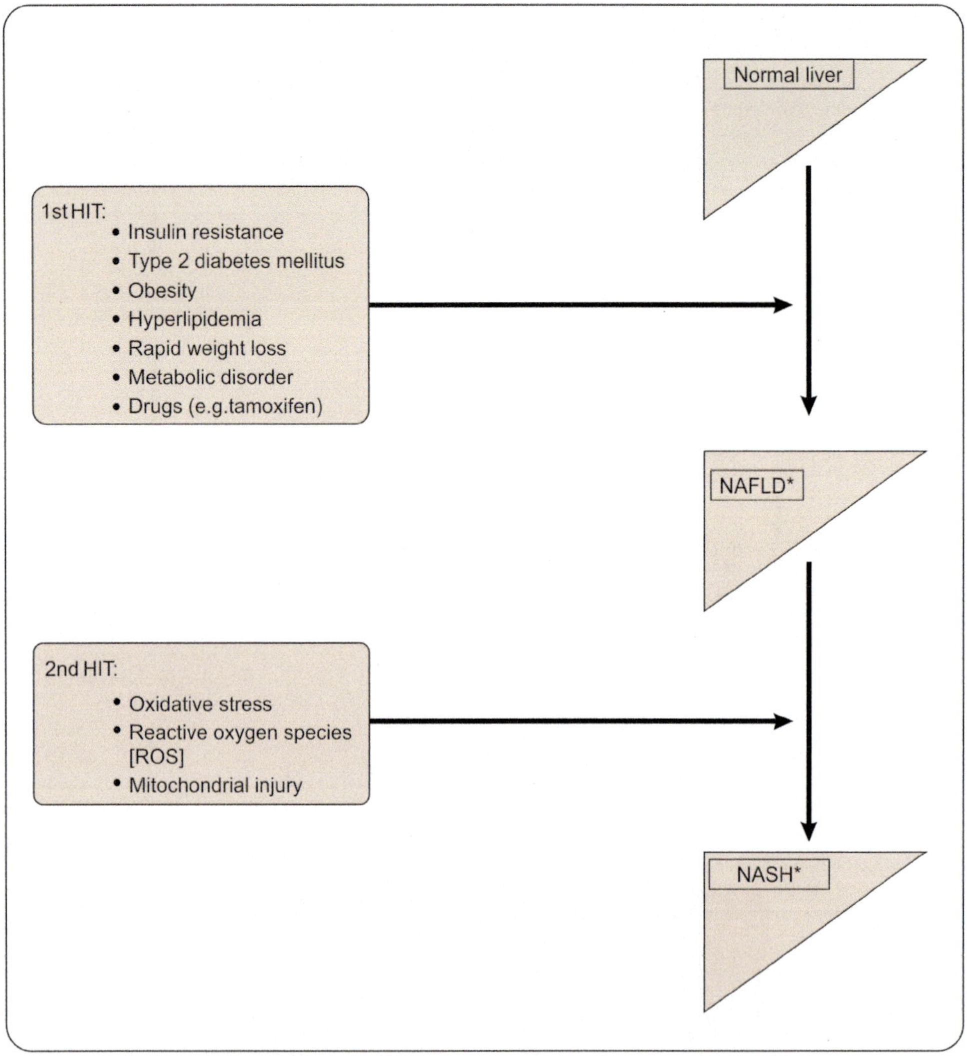

The pathogenesis of NAFLD is not entirely known, but a "2 Hit hypothesis" model has been proposed to describe it. The 2 Hits are:

- 1st Hit: Hepatic fat accumulation
- 2nd Hit: Oxidative stress on liver.

(*NAFLD: Nonalcoholic fatty liver disease and NASH: Nonalcoholic steatohepatitis).

What are the different pathologic stages in the progression of NAFLD?

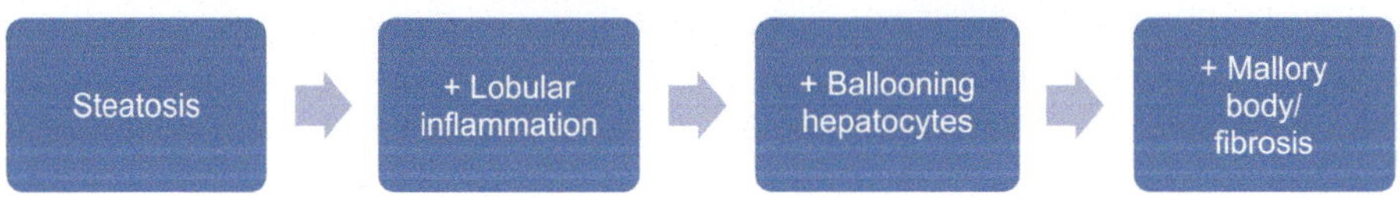

Further reading: NAFLD activity score (NAS score) and fibrosis staging:

Item	Score	Extent
Steatosis (Surface area involved by steatosis)	0 1 2 3	<5% (5–33)% (34–66)% >66%
Lobular inflammation (No. of focus per 200X)	0 1 2 3	No foci <2 foci 2–4 foci >4 foci
Hepatocyte ballooning	0 1 2	None Few cells Many cells/prominent ballooning
Fibrosis (Evaluated separately from NAS score)	0 1 2 3 4	None Perisinusoidal/periportal Perisinusoidal + periportal/portal Bridging fibrosis Cirrhosis

(A NAS score of 0–2: Not diagnostic of NASH; 3–4: Marginal and 5–8 is considered diagnostic of NASH).

What is the morphological classification of fatty liver and give some of the causes of each?

Morphological types	Description	Common causes
Macrovesicular fatty liver	Intracellular lipid droplets with diameter ≥ 25 μM, shifting the nucleus to the periphery, usually single	• Obesity • Type 2 diabetes mellitus • Alcohol • Steroids • Kwashiorkor • Wilson's disease
Microvesicular fatty liver	Intracellular droplets with diameter 3–5 μM, often multiple	• Acute fatty liver of pregnancy • Viral hepatitis • Drugs (Salicylate/ Tetracycline)

Describe the histology of fatty liver.

- Section showing histology of liver tissue with normal architectural pattern.
- Hepatocytes are showing large clear vacuoles in the cytoplasm (Fig. 3.5).
- Nucleus has been pushed to the periphery by the cytoplasmic vacuole, to give the hepatocytes a resemblance to signet-ring. So, this morphology is known as "*signet-ring appearance*".

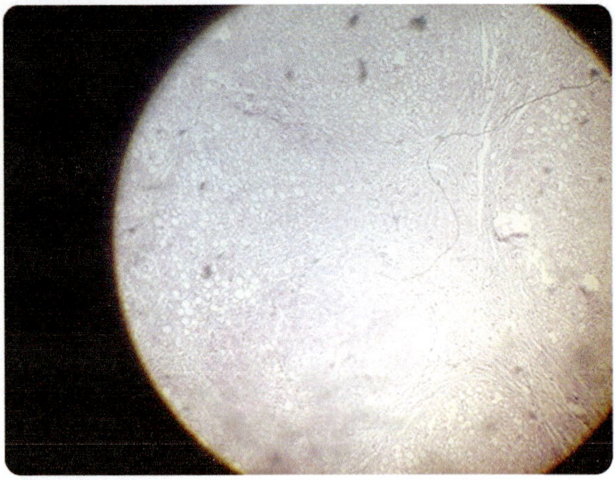

Fig. 3.5: Histology of fatty liver. Hepatocytes are showing clear vacuoles within the cytoplasm: Architectural pattern of tissue is preserved

Cirrhosis of liver

Description

This is a specimen of intact liver showing the following features (As shown in the following table) and the specimen is identified as "Cirrhosis of liver" (Figs 3.6A and B).

Features	Description
Color	Yellowish orange
Surface	Nodules of variable size alternating with depressed areas
Size	Shrunken
Margin	Sharp

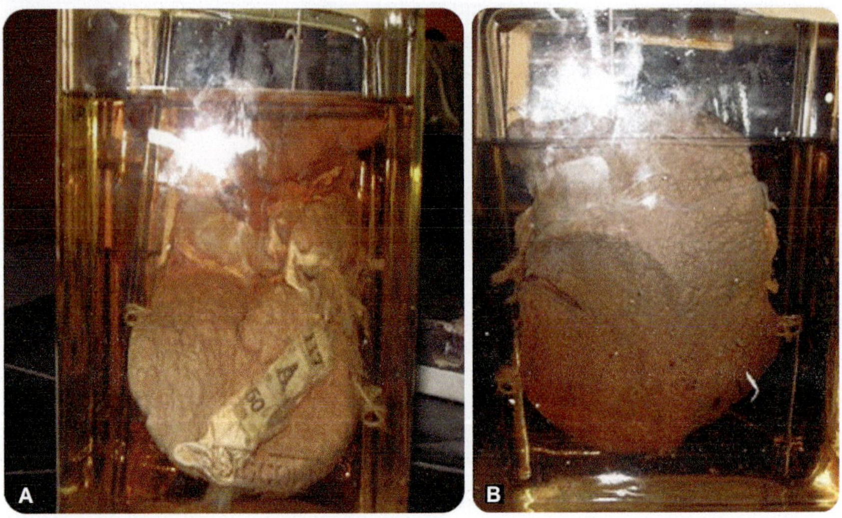

Figs 3.6A and B: Cirrhosis of liver. A. Front view and B. Back view

What do you mean by cirrhosis/define cirrhosis?

WHO definition of cirrhosis:
Cirrhosis is defined as a diffuse process characterized by fibrosis and the conversion of normal liver architecture into structurally abnormal nodules.

What are the criteria for diagnosis of cirrhosis?

1. **Parenchymal nodules**: They contain scattered foci of living hepatocytes surrounded by zones of fibrosis; resulting from repeated cycles of hepatocyte regeneration and scarring.

These are of two types:
   A. If the diameter is <3 mm, then it is called "Micronodule".
   B. If the diameter is >3 mm, then it is called "Macronodule".

   So, according to the presence of nodules, cirrhosis can be morphologically divided into 3 types:

   A. **Micronodular pattern**:
   - Abundant micronodules are found.
   - The striking feature is the regularity in the nodule size.
   - Generally they don't contain any normal structures within them (like portal tract/efferent vein, etc.).

   B. **Macronodular pattern**:
   - Abundant macronodules are found.
   - The nodule size is variable.
   - They may contain normal hepatic structures (portal tract/efferent vein, etc.).

   C. **Mixed pattern**:
   - When micronodules and macronodules are present in approximately equal proportions, the term "Mixed" is used.

2. **Bridging fibrous septa**: These are mainly of 2 types:
   A. Linking one portal tract to another
   B. Linking portal tracts with terminal hepatic veins.

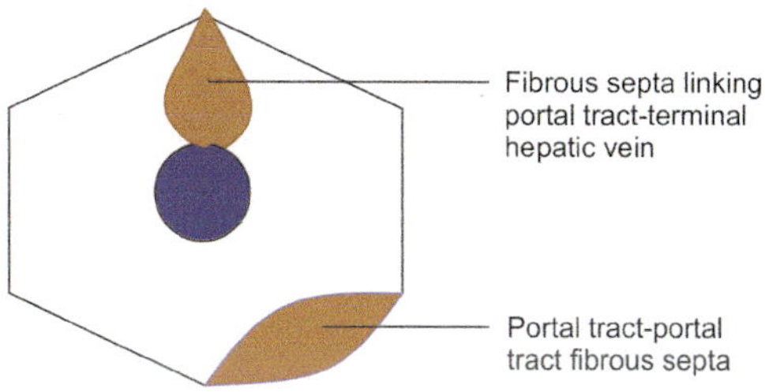

3. **Disorganization of the lobular architecture of the entire liver**: As cirrhosis is an irreversible and terminal stage of chronic liver diseases, it is characterized by diffuse involvement of the liver, comprising of:
   A. Diffuse parenchymal injury and necrosis
   B. Diffuse fibrosis.

What is the basis of nodule formation in cirrhosis?

Throughout the process of liver damage and fibrosis in the development of cirrhosis, the surviving hepatocytes are stimulated to regenerate and proliferate as spherical nodules within the confines of the fibrous septa.

What is the basis of depressions found in cirrhotic liver?

The alternating depressions occur due to contraction of fibrous bands and atrophy of hepatocytes.

Can you name some etiological factors associated with cirrhosis of liver?

Etiological association	*Etiological factors*
Established	• Viral hepatitis • Alcoholic and nonalcoholic fatty liver disease • Primary biliary cirrhosis • Secondary biliary cirrhosis • Metabolic disorders: – Wilson's disease – Hemochromatosis – α_1- antitrypsin deficiency, etc. • Drugs: – Methotrexate – α-methyldopa
Debatable	• Autoimmunity • Malnutrition • Schistosomiasis
Unknown	• Indian childhood cirrhosis • Cryptogenic cirrhosis

Here, we are discussing the pathogenesis of some of the important well-established etiological factors that are responsible for cirrhosis:

1. **Viral hepatitis (Type B, C, D)**: These viruses are responsible for cirrhosis of liver in a background of chronic hepatitis; which is associated more with hepatitis C virus; although hepatitis B and hepatitis D viruses (Hepatitis D is active only in the presence of Hepatitis B virus) cause a substantial number of liver cirrhosis.
2. **Alcoholic fatty liver disease (AFLD)/ Alcoholic steatohepatitis (ASH)**: Cirrhosis is the final and irreversible outcome. The successive stages are:

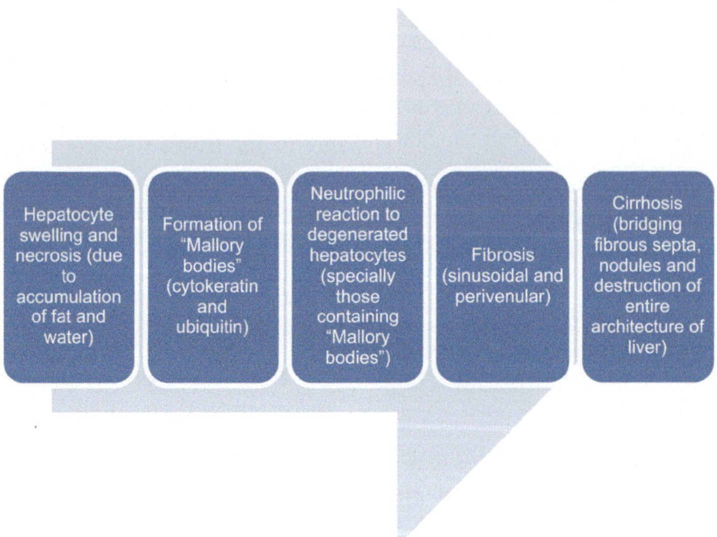

3. **Nonalcoholic fatty liver disease (NAFLD)**: It occurs in persons who don't consume alcohol. It should be remembered that the histological features of NASH (nonalcoholic steatohepatitis) are same as ASH (alcoholic steatohepatitis) and in both; cirrhosis is the final outcome.

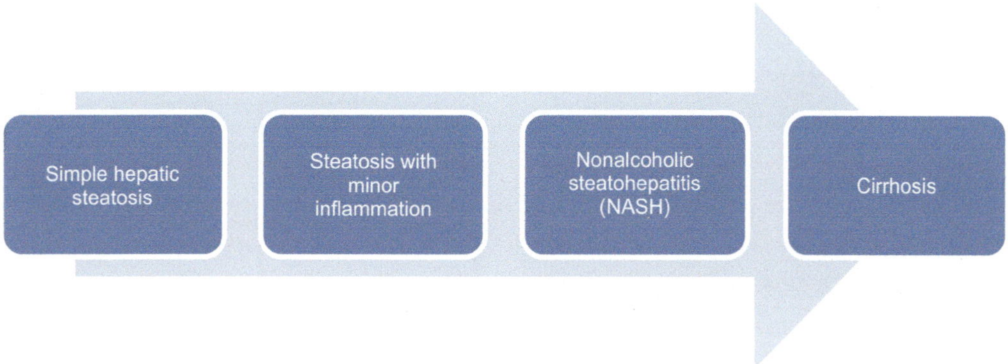

4. **Hemochromatosis**:
   It is of 2 types:
   i. Hereditary
   ii. Secondary.

Types of hemochromatosis	*Causes*
Hereditary hemochromatosis	Mutations in: • Transferrin receptor • Hepcidin
Secondary hemochromatosis/Hemosiderosis/ Secondary iron overload	• Transfusion • Long-term dialysis • Aplastic anemia • Sickle cell disease • Beta-thalassemia • Sideroblastic anemia • Chronic liver disease

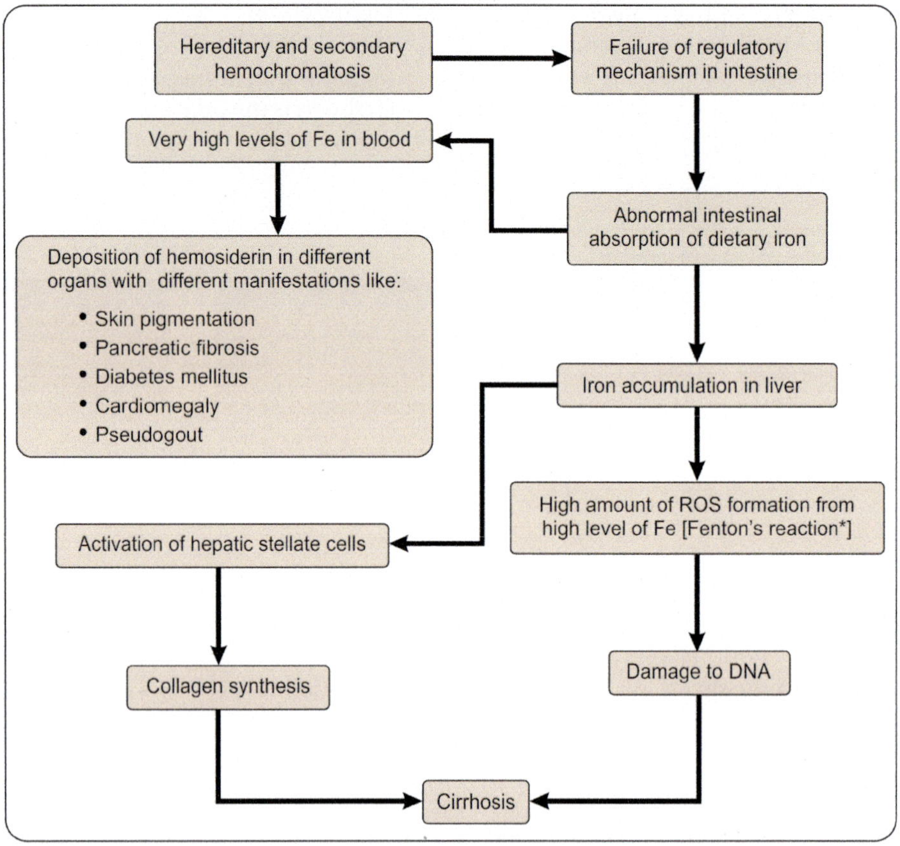

(* Fenton's reaction:

$$Fe^{++} + H_2O_2 \longrightarrow Fe^{+++} + OH^- + OH$$
$$Fe^{+++} + H_2O_2 \longrightarrow Fe^{++} + H^+ + OOH)$$

5. **Wilson's disease**:

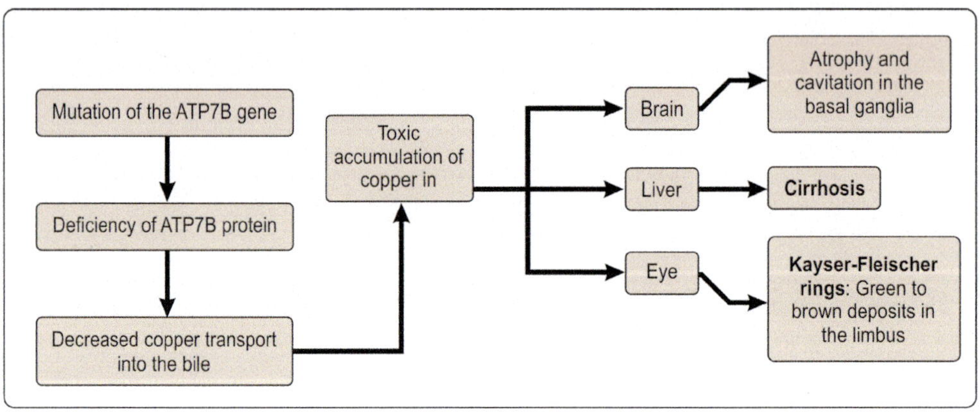

6. **α$_1$-antitrypsin deficiency** (Predominantly seen in children):

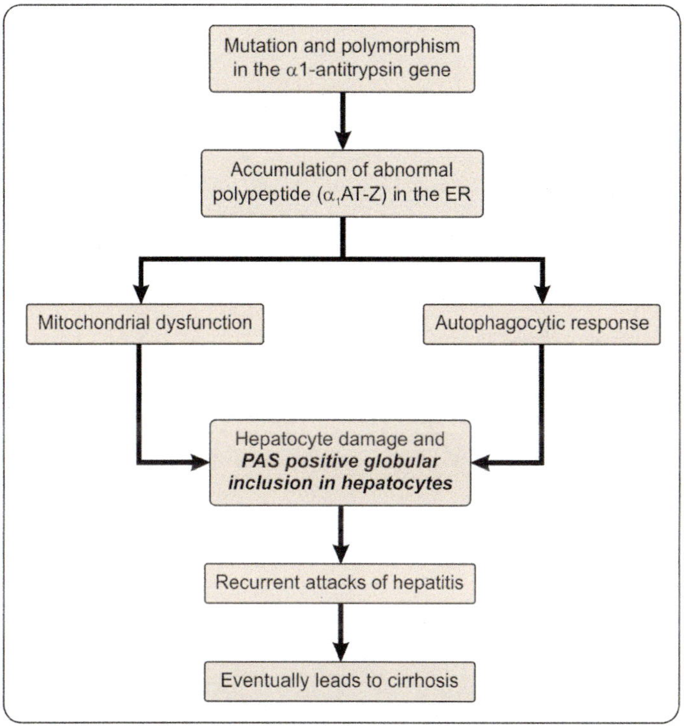

7. **Primary biliary cirrhosis (PBC)**:

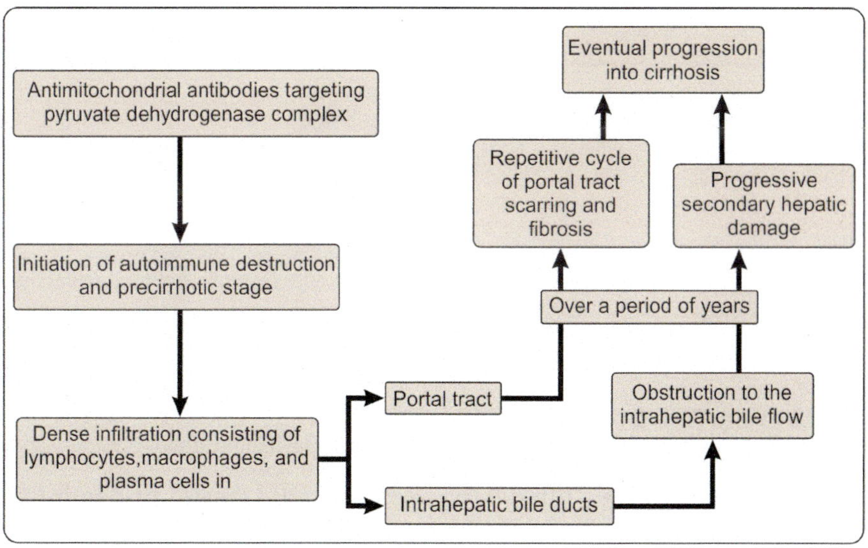

8. **Secondary biliary cirrhosis (SBC):**

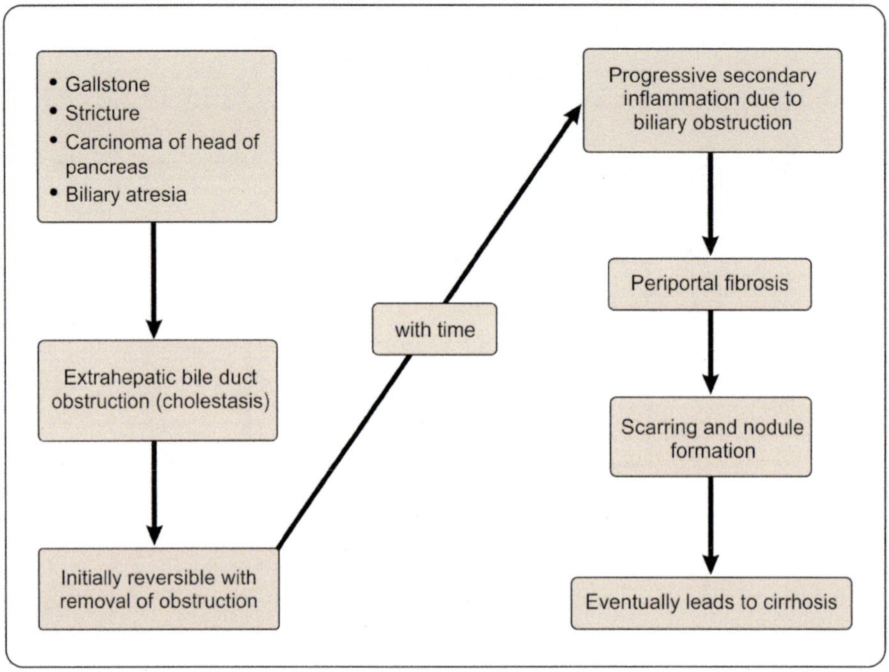

Mention the complications of cirrhosis.

Causes	*Complications*
Due to portal obstruction and portal hypertension	• Ascites • Splenomegaly • Esophageal varices/caput medusa
Due to hepatocyte damage	• Coagulation defect • Macrocytic anemia • Hypoproteinemia: Edema and ascites • Malignant transformation to hepatocellular carcinoma

What are the causes of bleeding in portal cirrhosis?

1. Due to portal hypertension, rupture of anastomotic vessels occurs.
2. Coagulation defect due to deficiency of coagulation factors.

What are the causes of death in portal cirrhosis?

1. Secondary infection
2. Hemorrhage
3. Hepatic coma
4. Acute pulmonary edema.

Metastatic carcinoma of liver

Description

- It is a specimen of cut section of liver showing multiple, large, and nodular growths.
- The nodules are yellowish white in color.
- Central parts of many nodules are depressed (umbilication).
- There are blackish areas of hemorrhage and areas of cystic changes.
  - So, the specimen is identified as "Metastatic carcinoma of liver" (Figs 3.7A and B).

Why this is not a specimen of cirrhosis?

Because in cirrhosis:
- The nodules are surrounded by fibrous bands.
- Nodules are smaller and never show umbilication.
- Usually no areas of hemorrhage/ necrosis are seen in cirrhosis.

Why this is not a specimen of hepatocellular carcinoma?

Because in hepatocellular carcinoma:
- The growth is usually solitary and massive.
- Umbilication is absent.
- Surrounding liver tissue is usually cirrhotic.

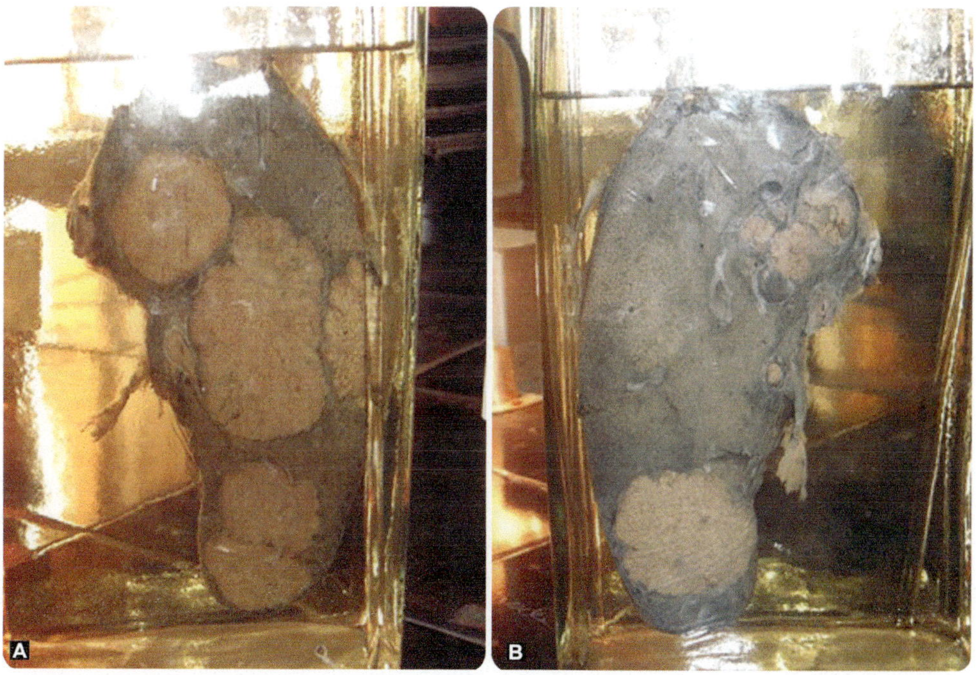

Figs 3.7A and B: Metastatic carcinoma of liver. A. Front view and B. Back view

What are the sources of metastasis in this specimen?

General route	*Description of spread*
Direct invasion from	• Gallbladder • Head of pancreas • Hepatic flexure of colon
Lymphatic spread from	• Stomach • Breast
From portal vein	• Stomach • Colorectal areas of gut (most common) • Small intestine
From hepatic artery	• Kidney • Bones • Uterus • Thyroid

CHAPTER

4

Kidney

Large white kidney

Description

- Kidney is enlarged
- Color of the specimen is pale/white
- Surface is smooth
- Capsule is thin.

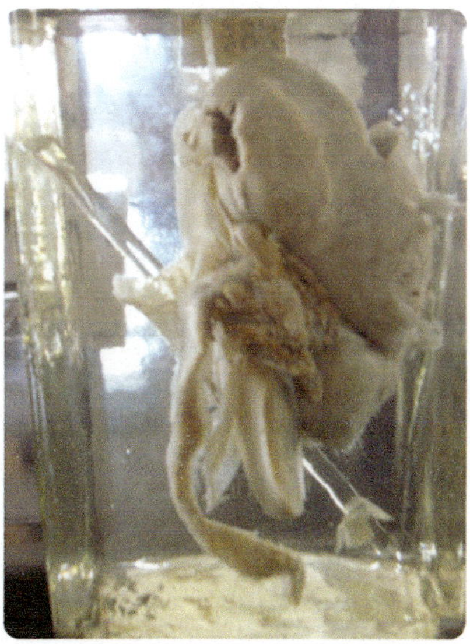

Fig. 4.1: Large white kidney

 – So, the above specimen is identified as "Large white kidney" (Fig. 4.1).

[Note: Capsule may easily be stripped off, consistency is soft.]

What are the common causes of large white kidney?

1. Rapidly progressing glomerulonephritis (RPGN): Most common cause.
2. Membranous glomerulonephritis.
3. Membranoproliferative glomerulonephritis.
4. Amyloid kidney.

Why is the kidney large and white?

- **Large**: Due to edema.
- **White**: Due to associated vascular compression.

Describe the histology of RPGN.

- The histologic picture is dominated by distinctive **crescents** (Fig. 4.2).
- Crescents are formed by proliferation of parietal cells and by migration of monocytes and macrophages into the urinary space.
- Eventually, most crescents undergo sclerosis.

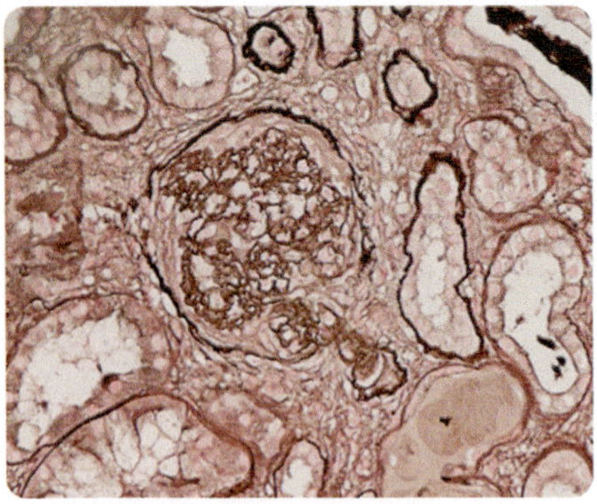

Fig. 4.2: Photomicrograph of a renal biopsy specimen showing crescent formation and tuft narrowing; Jones' stain. Reproduced under the permission of Dr Ramaswami, Nephrologist, Queensland, Australia

What is the role of fibrin in the formation of crescents in RPGN?

Fibrin strands are frequently prominent between the cellular layers in the crescents; and it is thought that the escape of fibrinogen into Bowman space and its conversion to fibrin are an important contributor to crescent formation.

What are the different types of RPGN? Give 1 example of each.

There are 3 types of RPGN:

Types of RPGN	Examples
Anti GBM antibody induced disease (Type 1)	Goodpasture syndrome
Immune complex mediated RPGN (Type 2)	Postinfectious glomerulonephritis
Pauci immune type RPGN (Type 3)	Wegener granulomatosis

What are the immunofluorescence findings of different types of RPGN?

Types of RPGN	Immunofluorescence findings
Anti GBM antibody induced disease (Type 1)	Linear deposits of IgG
Immune complex mediated RPGN (Type 2)	Granular immune deposits
Pauci immune type RPGN (Type 3)	Little/ no deposits of anti GBM antibodies/ immune complex

What is the danger of RPGN?

RPGN is associated with rapid deterioration of renal function and if not immediately, death from renal failure may occur within weeks to months.

Other important questions that may be asked from this point

What are the findings of light microscopy/ immunofluorescence/electron microscopy of poststreptococcal glomerulonephritis (PSGN).

Diagnostic procedures	Findings
Light microscopy	Enlarged and hypercellular glomeruli
Immunofluorescence	Granular deposits of IgG, IgM, and C_3 in the mesangium and along the GBM
Electron microscopy	Discrete electron-dense deposits on the epithelial side of the membrane

What is the cause of hypercellularity found in the light microscopy in case of poststreptococcal GN?

The hypercellularity in poststrep GN is caused by:

A. Proliferation of epithelial and mesangial cells
B. Infiltration of neutrophils and monocytes.

What are the manifestations of nephrotic syndrome and what are the causes of these manifestations?

Manifestations	*Causes*
Massive proteinuria (daily loss of protein is ≥3.5 gm)	Damage to the glomerular capillary walls resulting in increased permeability to plasma proteins
Hypoalbuminemia (plasma albumin level is <3 gm/dL)	Loss of large portions of albumin through the urine
Generalized edema	• Decreased colloid osmotic pressure (COP) of the blood with subsequent accumulation of fluid in the interstitial tissues • Sodium and water retention
Hyperlipidemia and lipiduria	• Increased synthesis of lipoproteins in the liver • Decreased catabolism of lipids

Name some genes which, when mutated, may lead to nephrotic syndrome?

Name of the gene	*Name of the coded protein*	*Name of the nephrotic syndrome*
NPHS1	Nephrin	Congenital nephrotic syndrome: Finnish type
NPHS2	Podosin	Steroid resistant nephrotic syndrome: Childhood onset

Name some common causes of nephrotic syndrome.

Causes	*Examples*
Primary glomerular diseases	• Minimal change disease • Focal segmental glomerulosclerosis (FSGS) • Membranous nephropathy • Membranoproliferative glomerulosclerosis* • IgA nephropathy
Systemic diseases	• Diabetes mellitus • SLE • Amyloidosis • Malignancy • Infections (mainly STDs like HIV, HBV, syphilis)

(* often has mixed nephritic/nephrotic syndrome)

What is the most frequent cause of nephrotic syndrome in children? What is its characteristic histological feature? Why the prognosis is usually good?

- Minimal change disease; it is commonly seen in children of 2–6 years of age.
- The most characteristic histological feature is diffuse effacement of foot processes of visceral epithelial cells (podocytes) in glomeruli, which is visible only in electron microscopy.
- The most striking feature is that the glomeruli in minimal change disease appear almost normal when seen in light microscopy.
- The prognosis is excellent because of its dramatic response to corticosteroid therapy.

What do you mean by focal segmental glomerulosclerosis (FSGS)?

- **Focal**: Only some of the glomeruli are involved.

- **Segmental**: In the affected glomeruli, only a portion of the capillary is involved.
- **Glomerulosclerosis**: The change in the glomeruli is mainly sclerosis.

What do you mean by hyalinosis and sclerosis?

- **Hyalinosis**: Extracellular deposition/ entrapment of plasma proteins into the glomerular structures.
- **Sclerosis**: Accumulation of extracellular collagenous matrix (ECM) in the mesangium/ capillary loops.
  - They are common features of FSGS.

Shortly tell the pathogenesis and specific findings in membranous nephropathy and membranoproliferative glomerulonephritis (MPGN).

Diseases	Pathogenesis	Light microscopy	Fluorescence microscopy	Electron microscopy
Membranous nephropathy	Immune complex formation in glomerulus	Uniform and diffuse thickening of glomerular capillary wall	Granular deposits (C_3 + IgG)	Subepithelial electron-dense deposits
MPGN type 1	Immune complex in glomerulus; activation of both classical and alternative complement pathways	The large and hypercellular glomeruli show "lobular" appearance due to the proliferating mesangial cells and increased proliferation of mesangial matrix	Granular deposits (C_3 + IgG; C1q + C_4)	Subendothelial deposits
MPGN type 2	Activation of alternative complement pathway only	Glomerular capillary wall shows "Tram track appearance", due to duplication of GBM	Granular/linear deposits (C_3±IgG)	Dense deposits in the GBM

Name the characteristic changes in the diabetic nephropathy.

1. Glomerular lesions:
   a. Capillary basement membrane thickening.
   b. Diffuse mesangial sclerosis.
   c. Nodular glomerulosclerosis (with fibrin caps and capsular drops).
2. Hyaline arteriolosclerosis of the afferent and efferent arteriole.
3. Acute pyelonephritis (papillary necrosis).

What is the similarity of IgA nephropathy and renal manifestation of Henoch-Schönlein purpura? What is the conclusion from this similarity?

- In both of the diseases, IgA is deposited in the glomerular mesangium.
- This has led to the concept that IgA nephropathy and HS purpura are both manifestations of the same disease.

Name the glomerulopathy most commonly seen in patients of HIV.

- Collapsing glomerulopathy; it is a morphologic variant of FSGS (focal segmental glomerulosclerosis).
- The pathogenesis of HIV-related FSGS is thought to be due to infection of glomerular and tubular cells by HIV.

Granular contracted kidney

Description

- Size of kidney is grossly reduced.
- Surface is finely granular.

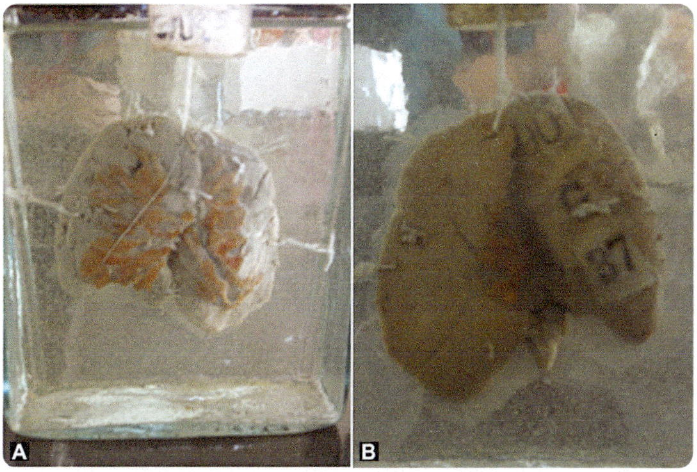

Figs 4.3A and B: Granular contracted kidney. A. Front view and B. Back view

- Capsule is adherent and consistency is firm.
  - So, the specimen is identified as "Granular contracted kidney" (Figs 4.3A and B).

What are the main causes of granular contracted kidney?

1. Chronic glomerulonephritis: Most common cause.
2. Benign nephrosclerosis
3. Chronic pyelonephritis
4. Less common causes:
   Terminal stages of:
   - Amyloid/myeloma kidney
   - Diabetic nephropathy.

What are the main causes of chronic glomerulonephritis?

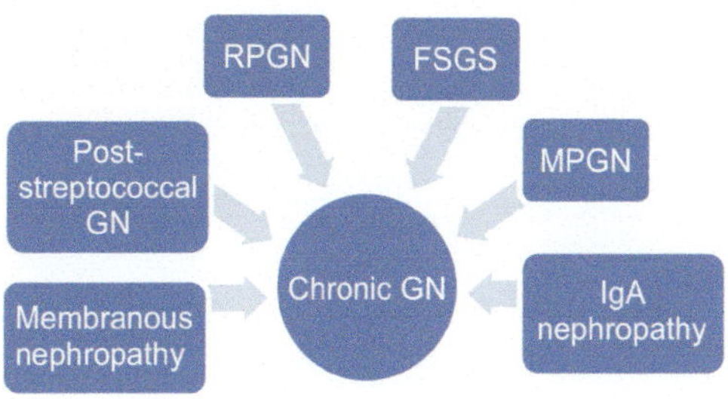

Describe the morphology of chronic GN.

Gross morphology:

- The kidneys are symmetrically contracted.
- They have diffusely granular cortical surfaces.
- On section, the cortex is thinned.
- There is an increase in peripelvic fat.

Histology:

The glomerular histology depends on the stage of the disease.

Stages	*Histology*
Early stage	The glomeruli still show evidence of the primary disease (as given in the causes of the chronic GN above)
Late stage	Obliteration of glomeruli transforms the glomeruli into acellular eosinophilic masses, consisting of a combination of: 1. Hyaline 2. Collagen 3. Trapped plasma proteins 4. Increased mesangial matrix (Fig. 4.4)

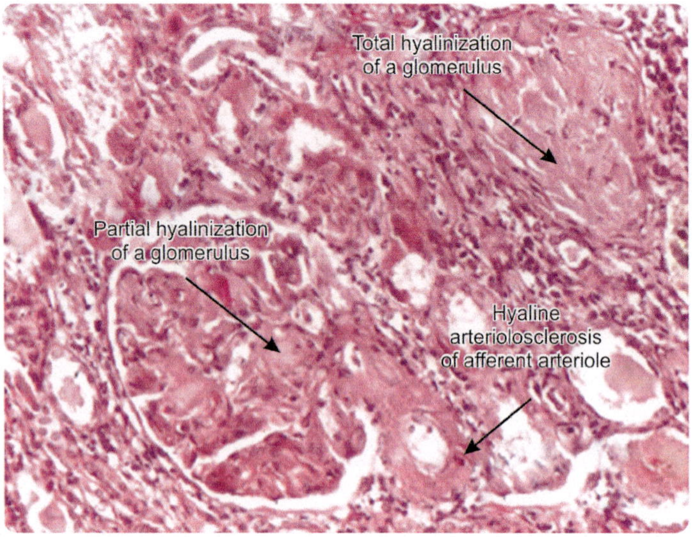

Fig. 4.4: Histology of late stage chronic glomerulonephritis. Reproduced under the permission of Dr Mihai Danciu, Gr T Popa University of Medicine and Pharmacy, Iasi, Romania

What is the association between chronic GN and hypertension?

- Most patients with chronic GN are hypertensive.
- Sometimes the dominant clinical manifestations are cerebral/cardio-vascular.
- Because hypertension is an usual associated condition of chronic glomerulonephritis, the following histological features may be seen:

1. Hyaline arteriolosclerosis (Fig. 4.4)
2. Marked atrophy of associated tubules.

Describe the important urinary findings in such a case.

What is the treatment of chronic GN?

- There are very few options left as the kidneys are slowly progressing to renal insufficiency and the patients may die of uremia in upcoming years.
- The only options are:
  a. Continued dialysis
  b. Renal transplant.
- But in patients with long-term dialysis, certain risks are there like:
  a. Acquired cystic disease.
  b. Increased number of renal adenomas and carcinomas.
- So, renal transplant seems to be the only option.

Parameters	Description
Physical	• Volume: Large • Color: Pale • Transparency: Clear • Specific gravity: Low and fixed (1010)— Isothenuria
Chemical	Mild to moderate proteinuria
Microscopical	Granular cast present

Hydronephrosis

Description

- The kidney is enlarged.
- Cut section shows multiple cystic cavities which are communicating with renal pelvis.
- Wall of cyst is very thin and devoid of congestion.
- Pelvis of ureter is dilated.
  - So, the specimen is identified as "Hydronephrosis" (Figs 4.5A and B).

Why this is not a specimen of polycystic kidney?

Because in polycystic kidney, the cysts do not communicate with renal pelvis.

Why this is not a specimen of pyelonephritis?

Because in pyelonephritis, the cyst walls are inflamed and congested.

What is hydronephrosis?

Hydronephrosis is described as dilation of the renal pelvis and calyces associated with progressive atrophy of the kidney due to obstruction to the outflow of urine (Figs 4.6A and B).

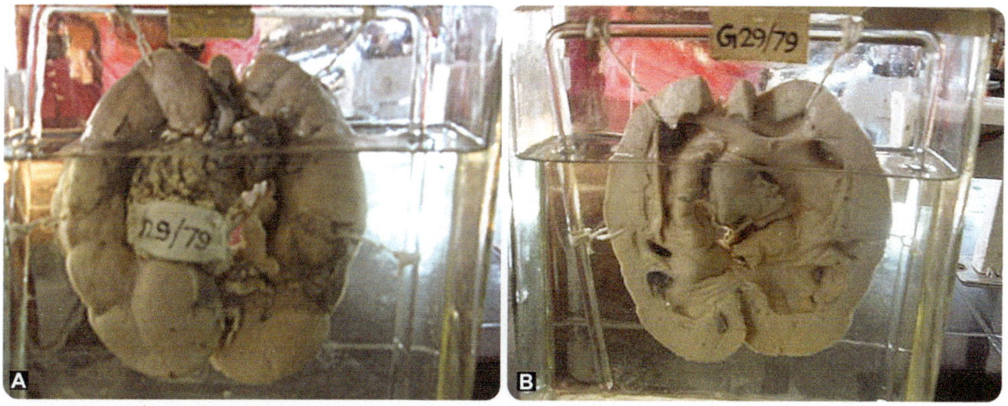

Figs 4.5A and B: Hydronephrosis. A. Front view and B. Back view

Name some causes of hydronephrosis.

Locations	*Causes*
Pelvis	• Calculi • Tumors
Ureter—Intrinsic causes	• Calculi • Tumors • Clot • Sloughed papillae inflammation
Ureter—Extrinsic causes	• Cervical tumors • Retroperitoneal fibrosis
Bladder	• Calculi • Tumors • Neurogenic bladder
Prostate	• Benign nodular hyperplasia of prostate • Prostatic carcinoma • Prostatitis

Describe the pathogenesis of hydronephrosis.

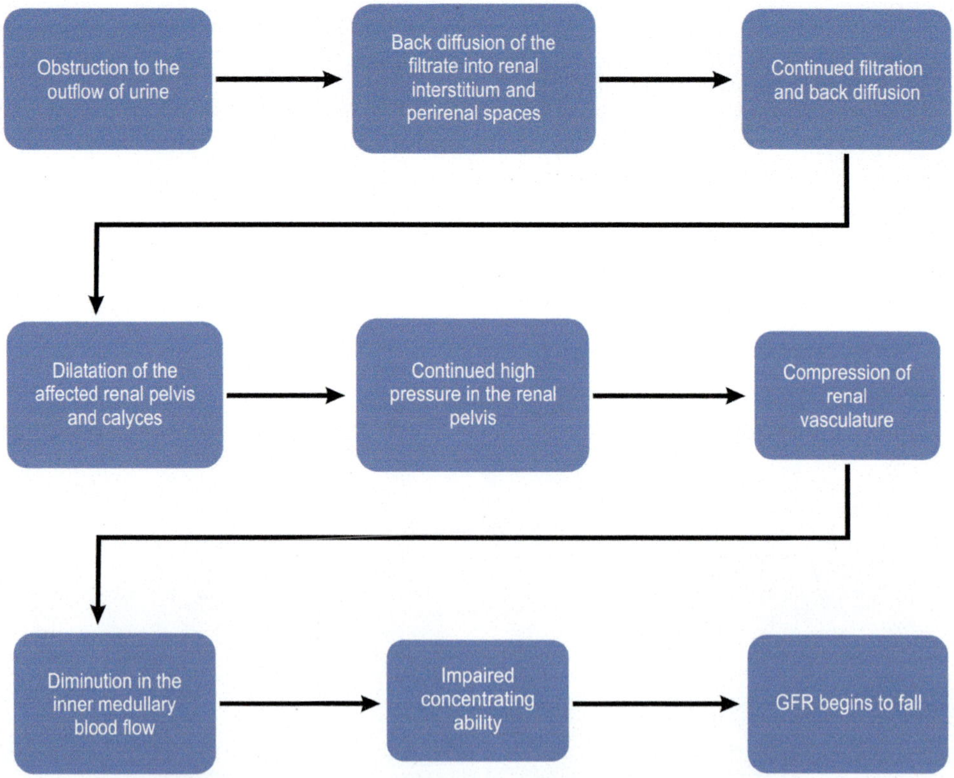

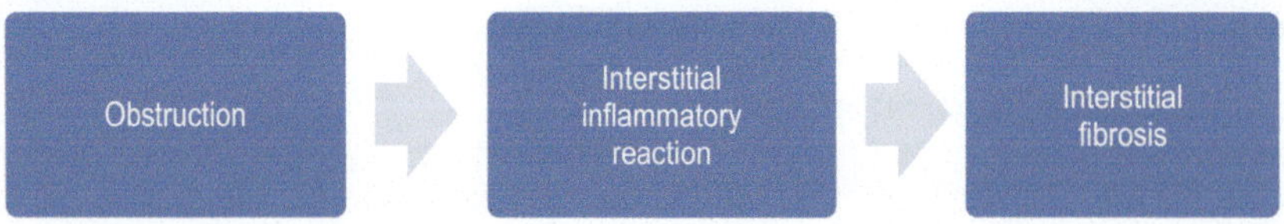

Describe the morphological changes seen in hydronephrosis.

Introduction:

- The kidney may be slightly to massively enlarged (depending on the degree and the duration of the obstruction).

Types of obstruction	*Effects on glomerular filtration*
Subtotal or intermittent	• Glomerular filtration is not suppressed • Progressive dilation of renal pelvis ensues
Sudden and complete	• Glomerular filtration is reduced • Mild dilation of the pelvis and calyces • Atrophy of the renal parenchyma

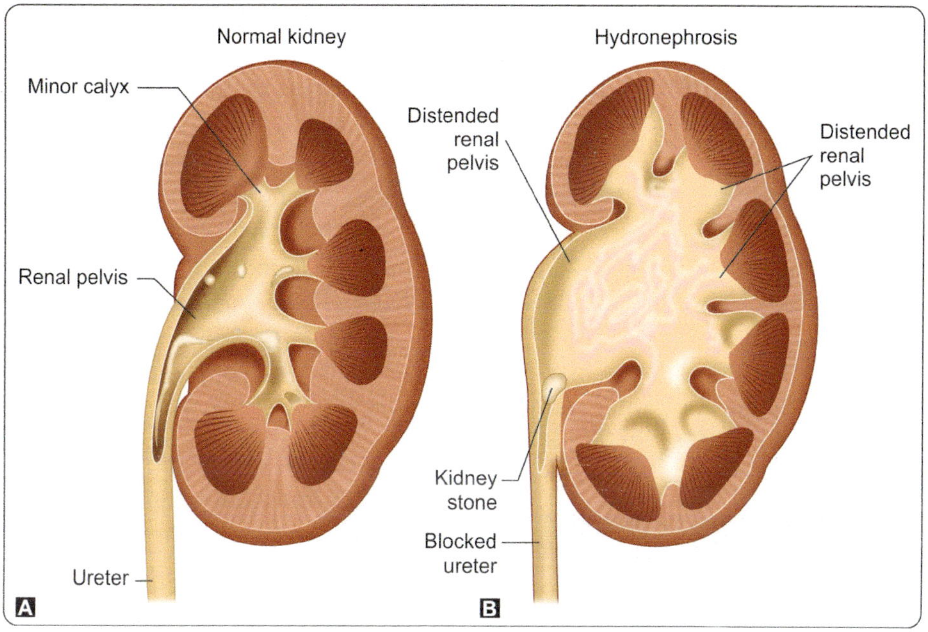

Figs 4.6A and B: A. Normal kidney and B. Kidney with hydronephrosis. Note the distension of the renal pelvis on the right kidney. In this illustration, the distension is caused by a kidney stone blocking the ureter, causing the urine to back diffuse to the renal pelvis

Morphological changes: Compare with the pathogenesis of hydronephrosis.

Duration of obstruction	*Morphological changes*
Acute onset	Dilation of the pelvis and calyces with interstitial inflammation
Chronic onset	Cortical tubular atrophy with diffuse interstitial fibrosis
Advanced case	The kidney is transformed into a thin-walled cystic structure with: • Extensive parenchymal atrophy • Total obliteration of the pyramids • Thinning of the cortex

Polycystic kidney disease

Description

- The kidney is enlarged.
- Multiple small/large cysts are projecting on the surface in bunch.
- In between the cysts, the kidney tissues are white and atrophied.
- **All the cysts fail to communicate with the renal pelvis**.
- Renal pelvis is usually not dilated.
- When the cysts are cut in section, they show multiple cavities which contain viscid/clear fluid. It may be black due to hemorrhage within the cysts.
  - So, the specimen is identified as "Polycystic kidney disease" (Fig. 4.7).

Name some of the diseases where renal cysts are found.

1. Simple renal cyst
2. Polycystic kidney disease:
   a. ADPKD (Autosomal dominant polycystic kidney disease).
   b. ARPKD (Autosomal recessive polycystic kidney disease).

3. Multicystic renal dysplasia
4. Medullary cystic disease
5. Glomerulocystic disease
6. Extraparenchymal renal cyst
7. Dialysis associated cystic disease.

Describe the pathogenesis of polycystic kidney diseases in brief.

1. Adult onset/autosomal dominant polycystic kidney disease (ADPKD):

Normal physiology:

- Each renal tubular epithelial cell contains a single nonmotile primary cilium, which projects into the tubular lumen.

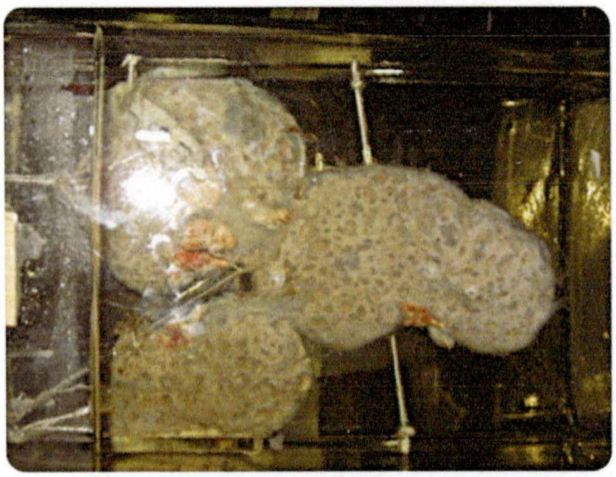

Fig. 4.7: Polycystic kidney disease

- This cilium senses external mechanical signals (e.g.: fluid flow).
- In response to these signals, these cilia regulate Ca^{++} ion flux.
- PKD1 and PKD2 genes translate 2 distinct proteins named polycystin 1 and polycystin 2, which are located in the cilium; possibly regulating the signal transduction (by Ca^{++}) and ultimately, growth and differentiation of tubular epithelial cells.

In ADPKD:

- In ADPKD, either the gene PKD1 or PKD2 is mutated, resulting in mutated polycystin 1/polycystin 2 production.
- So the mechanical sensation and signal transduction mechanism by the cilia are altered; leading to high levels of Ca^{++} influx into the cell and subsequent unregulated growth and differentiation of tubular epithelial cells; eventually leading to cyst development and enlargement of the cyst.

The possible mechanism for cyst formation is:

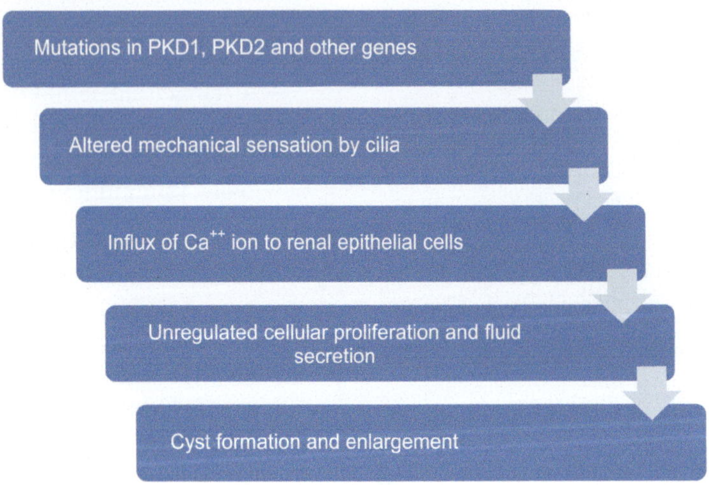

2. Childhood onset/autosomal recessive polycystic kidney disease (ARPKD):

- In most cases, the disease is caused by mutations of the PKHD1 gene which encodes another protein named "Fibrocystin".
- Fibrocystin is thought to be a cell surface receptor responsible for differentiation of both collecting duct and biliary tract.
- So mutation in this "Double function" gene leads to the characteristic clinical scenario of:
  a. Presence of cysts in cortex and medulla
  b. Presence of cysts in liver, associated with hepatic fibrosis.

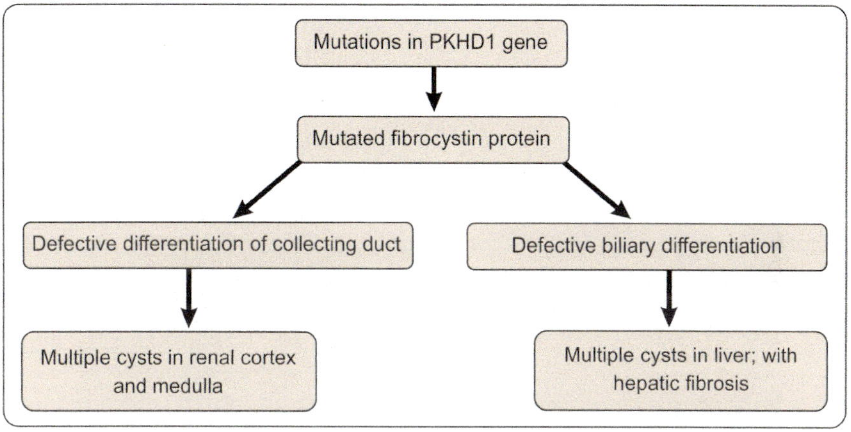

Tell some important morphological features of ADPKD and ARPKD.

Morphological features	*ADPKD/Adult PKD*	*ARPKD/ Childhood PKD*
Gross appearance	The kidneys are usually bilaterally enlarged and external surface appears to be composed solely of a mass of cysts, upto 3–4 cm in diameter, with no intervening parenchyma	• The kidneys are enlarged and have a smooth external surface • Only a cut section reveals numerous small cysts in the cortex and medulla
Prominent microscopic finding	Microscopic examination reveals functioning nephrons dispersed between the cysts	Microscopic examination reveals **dilation of all collecting tubules**
Cell of origin	The cysts arise from the tubules throughout the nephron and therefore have variable lining epithelia	The cysts have a uniform lining of cuboidal cells, reflecting their origin from the collecting ducts
Involvement of liver	About 40% of the patients have one to several cysts in the liver (polycystic liver disease) that are usually asymptomatic	In almost all cases the liver has cysts associated with portal fibrosis (congenital hepatic fibrosis). Such patients may develop **portal hypertension with splenomegaly**

Name one cystic disease of kidney where most of the cysts are located at the junction of renal cortex and medulla.

Medullary cystic disease.

Name one cystic disease of kidney which may progress into renal cell carcinoma (RCC).

Dialysis associated cystic disease.

Renal cell carcinoma

Description

- This is a nephrectomy specimen showing the cut surface of a kidney with a yellowish orange growth diffusely involving almost the whole of the kidney.
- This growth has extended inside the cut surface and it has invaded the renal calyces.
- Extensive area of hemorrhage and necrosis is being seen.
  - So, this specimen is identified as "Renal cell carcinoma" (Figs 4.8A and B).

What are the major types of renal cell carcinoma?

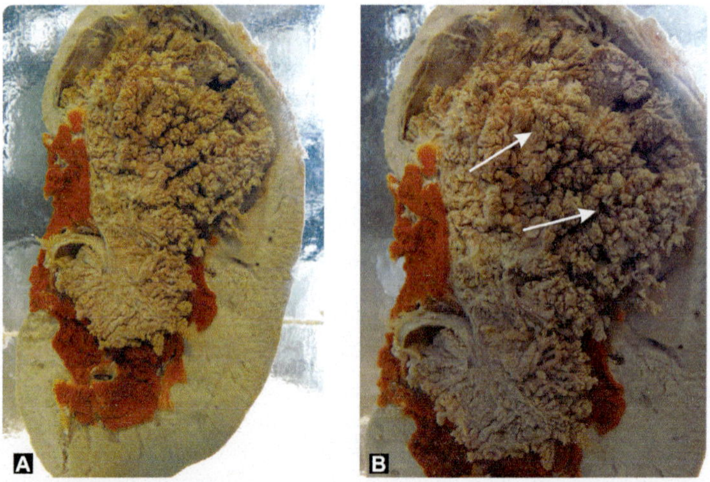

Figs 4.8A and B: A specimen of kidney with renal cell carcinoma showing extensive invasion of renal calyces (arrows) and areas of hemorrhage

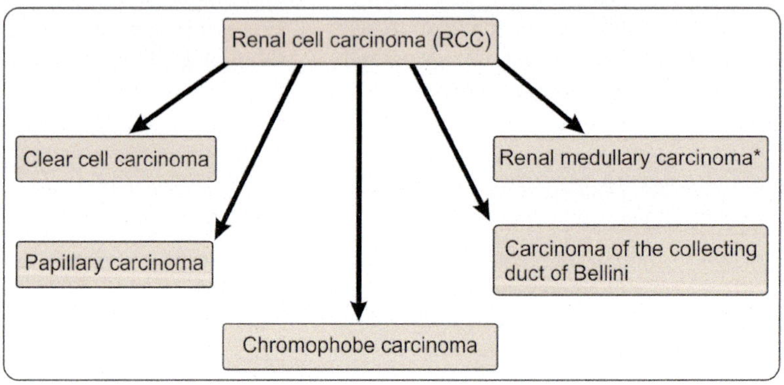

(*Rare)

Describe the major histological features of some important types of RCC.

RCC subtype	Incidence	Development	Growth pattern	Morphology
Clear cell	75%	Solitary, rarely multifocal or bilateral	Solid, tubular, cystic	Clear cytoplasm; cells with eosinophilic cytoplasm occasionally
Papillary	10%	Multifocal, bilateral or solitary	Tubulopapillary, solid	Type 1 (basophilic) or type 2 (eosinophilic)
Chromophobe	5%	Solitary	Solid	Pale or eosinophilic granular cytoplasm, usually with a perinuclear halo
Collecting duct of Bellini	1%	Solitary	Irregular channels	Eosinophilic cytoplasm

Can you name some genes associated with RCC?

- Clear cell carcinoma is identified by specific deletion of chromosome 3p and mutation of the VHL gene. Other changes are duplication of the chromosome band 5q22, deletion of chromosome 6q, 8p, 9p and 14q.
- Papillary carcinoma is associated most commonly with trisomies of chromosomes 3q, 7, 8, 12, 16, 17 and loss of chromosome Y.

What are the common paraneoplastic syndromes associated with RCC?

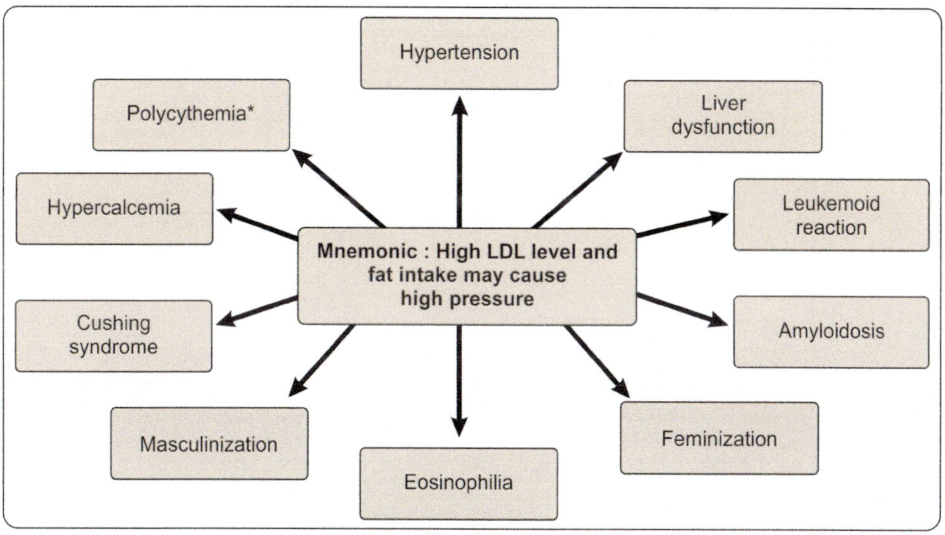

(* Polycythemia is the most common paraneoplastic syndrome associated with RCC; it is caused by a high amount of erythropoietin production by the tumor).

What are the classical diagnostic features of RCC?

1. Palpable mass
2. Costovertebral pain
3. Painless hematuria.

Define hematuria.

Hematuria is usually defined as >5 RBCs per high-power field in the urinary sediment.

What is the significance of pain associated with hematuria?

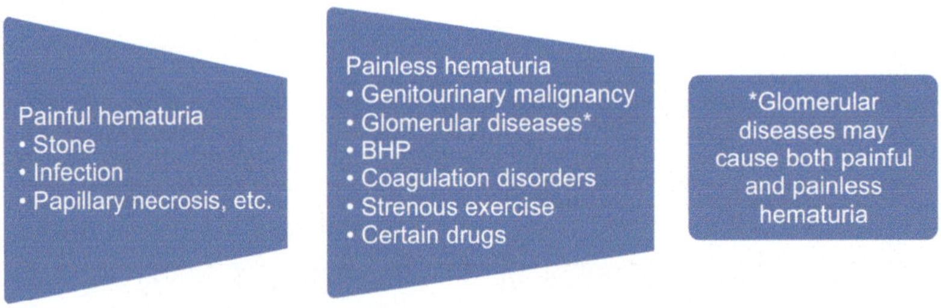

How do you confirm a diagnosis of cancer as a cause of painless hematuria?

30% of the patients with painless hematuria are found to have a malignancy (most commonly bladder cancer).

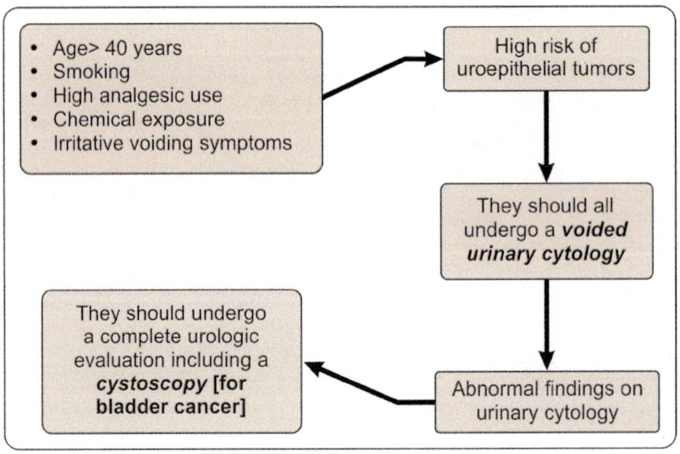

What are the common metastatic sites for RCC?

It should be mentioned that RCC, being an aggressive tumor, presents with distal metastasis in 1/4th of patients at the time of diagnosis. The common sites for metastasis are:

- Lungs and mediastinum
- Bone
- Liver
- Lymph nodes
- Adrenal gland
- Brain.

CHAPTER

5

Male Genital System

Carcinoma penis

Description

It is a specimen of penis with a large cauliflower-like fungating mass having rolled out and everted margin. The surface of growth is ulcerated.

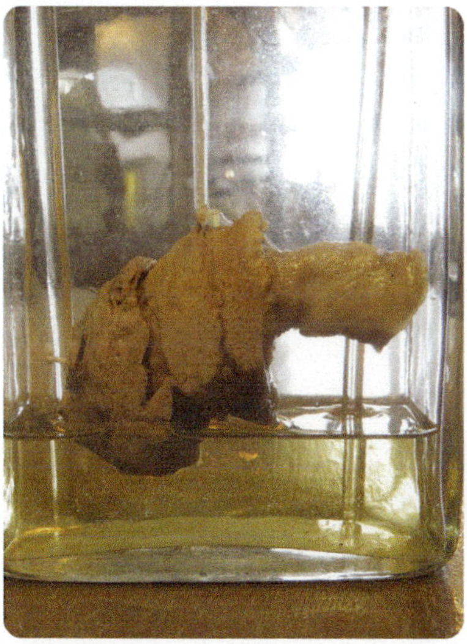

Fig. 5.1: Carcinoma penis. The specimen of penis is showing large cauliflower-like growth at coronal sulcus of the glans penis

- So, the specimen is identified as "Carcinoma penis" (Fig. 5.1).

What are the common sites of origin of carcinoma penis?

In decreased order of frequency

1. Glans penis: Most common
2. Frenulum
3. Prepuce.

What are the common macroscopic types of carcinoma penis?

Types	*Description*
Papillary	Produces cauliflower-like fungating mass
Flat	Produces epithelial thickening and eventually progresses into development of an ulcerative lesion

What is the major histologic type?

Squamous cell carcinoma.

What are the predisposing conditions?

1. Phimosis (when the orifice of the prepuce is too small to permit its normal retraction, the condition is designated as phimosis).

2. Chronic balanitis (Inflammation of the glans penis).
3. HPV type 16 infection.
4. Cigaret smoking.

What is the age of affected people?

Usually between 40 and 70.

What are the premalignant lesions?

1. Bowen's disease
2. Bowenoid papulosis.

What are the modes of spread?

Squamous cell carcinoma of penis is a slow growing and locally invasive carcinoma; disseminated metastasis is extremely uncommon.

Prognosis largely depends on the presence/absence of inguinal lymph node metastasis.

Mode of spread	Description
Local spread	• Infiltration of erectile tissue
Lymphatic spread	• In inguinal lymph node • Distal metastasis is uncommon

Seminoma testis

Description

It is a specimen showing a cut surface of testis which is:
- Homogeneous
- Lobulated
- Gray-white in color
- Devoid of hemorrhage and necrosis.
  - So, the specimen is identified as "Seminoma testis" (Fig. 5.2).

Describe the genetic abnormalities in seminoma testis.

- Seminomas are the most common type of germ cell tumor.
- Seminomas contain an isochromosome 12p.

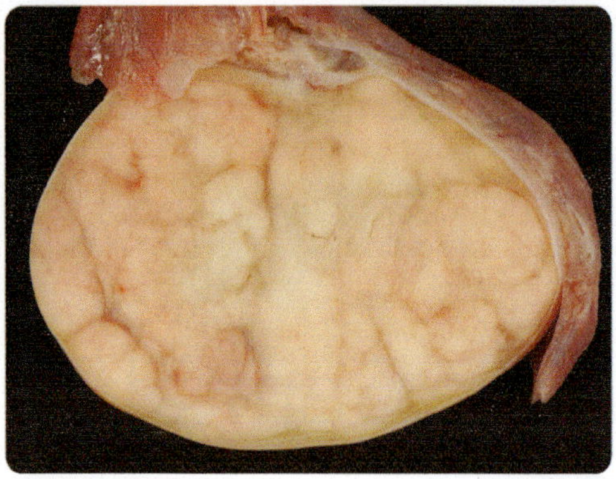

Fig. 5.2: Seminoma testis. A specimen of testis is cut open to show gray-white colored multilobulated tumor. Courtesy of Ed. Uthman, MD, Texas

- Some of the tumors have c-KIT activating mutations.

Describe the morphology of seminoma testis.

- Microscopically the typical seminoma is composed of:
  - Sheets of uniform cells divided into poorly differentiated lobules by

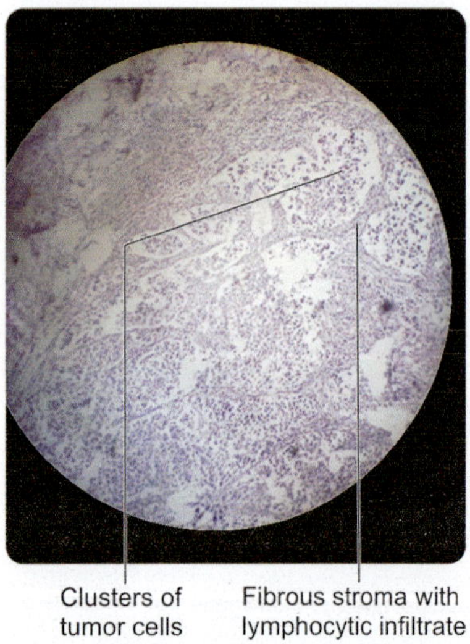

Fig. 5.3: Testicular seminoma, showing a prominent lymphocytic infiltrate in the fibrous stroma separating the clusters of tumor cells

delicate fibrous septa containing a prominent lymphocytic infiltrate (Fig. 5.3).

- The classic seminoma cell is large and have:
  - A distinct cell membrane.
  - A clear/watery cytoplasm (because of abundant glycogen).
  - A large central nucleus with 1–2 prominent nucleoli.

Benign hypertrophy of prostate/ benign prostatic hyperplasia

Description

It is a specimen of prostate gland showing:

- Enlargement of the gland
- Presence of large, fairly discrete nodules on the periurethral region of prostate.
  - So, the specimen is diagnosed as benign hypertrophy of prostate(Fig. 5.4).

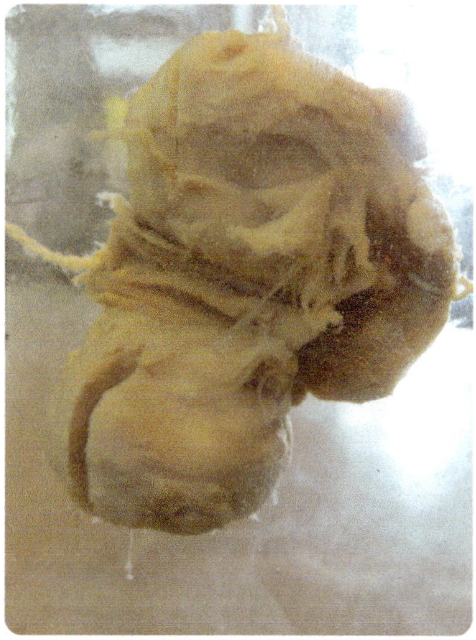

Fig. 5.4: Benign hypertrophy of prostate: Enlargement of both lateral lobes, cut section showing vague nodularity. Capsule intact

Describe the nodules found in BHP.

- The early nodules are composed almost entirely of *stromal cells.*
- The late nodules are predominantly composed of *epithelial cells.*

Why the diagnosis of BHP can't be made by needle biopsy?

1. Nodules characteristic of BHP usually originates from the **transition zone** of the prostate gland.
2. Needle biopsies cannot typically sample the transition zone.
3. The histology of glandular or mixed glandular-stromal nodules of BHP cannot be appreciated in limited samples.

Describe the pathogenesis of BHP.

Normal physiology:

- There are 2 important types of cells within prostate:
  A. Stromal cells
  B. Epithelial cells.
- The activation of testosterone into dihydrotestosterone (DHT) takes place within the stromal cells of prostate by the enzyme type 2 5α- reductase, which is present only within the stromal cells (not within the epithelial cells).
- After activation, DHT translocates into the nucleus of both epithelial

Type of nodules	Cell of origin	Morphology	Consistency	Color	Exude fluid?
Early	Stromal cells	Fibromuscular	Tough	Pale-gray	No
Late	Epithelial cells	Glandular	Soft	Yellow-pink	Yes; milky white fluid

cells and stromal cells and attaches to the androgen receptors; then the downstream activity results in growth and differentiation of both types of cells.

In BHP:

Several theories have been proposed to describe the pathogenesis of BHP. These include:

- An increase in the level of DHT; leading to increased cell growth.
- Reactivation of stem cells in resulting benign enlargement of prostate.
- Unregulated Stromal–epithelial interaction (Fig. 5.5).

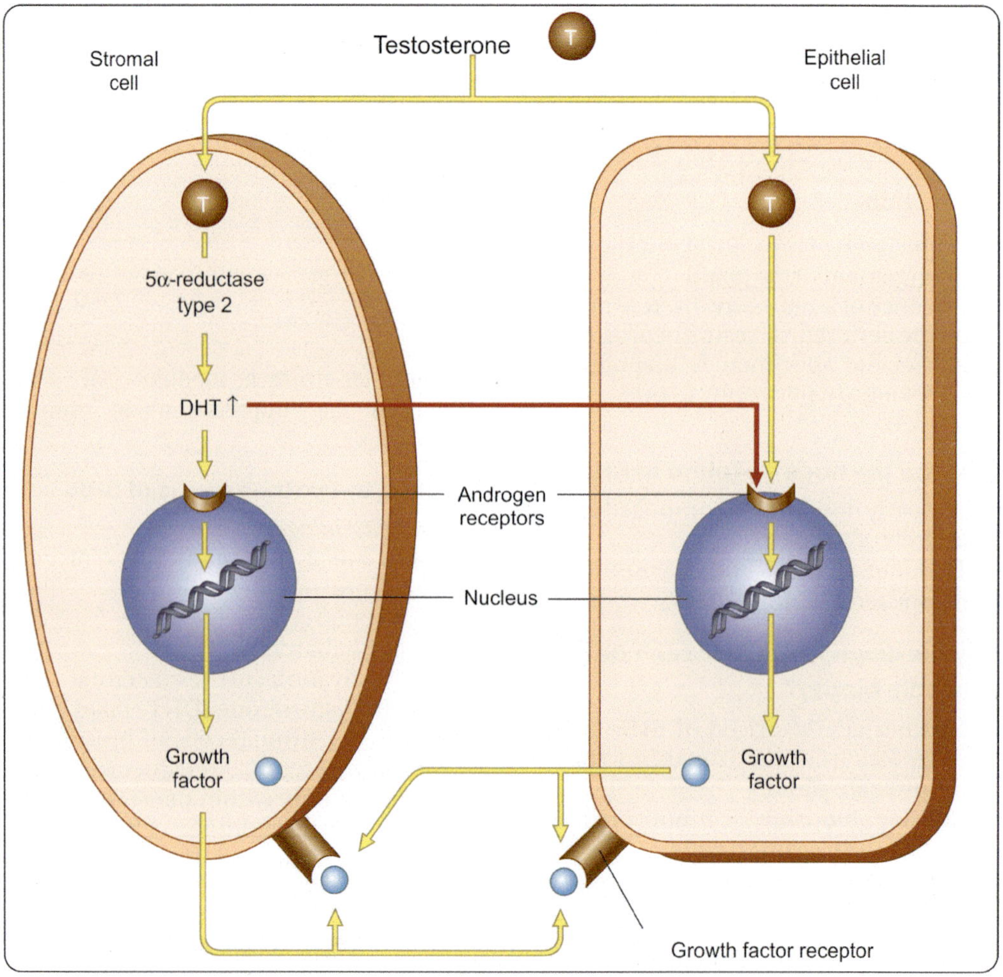

Fig. 5.5: Pathogenesis of BHP

What are the sequelae of BHP?

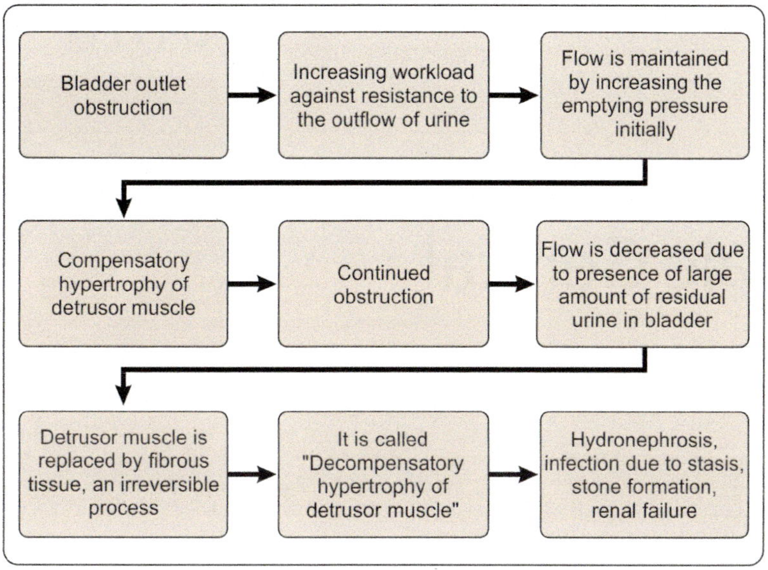

Can you name some treatment options for BHP?

1. Pharmacological:
   a. Type 2 5α-reductase inhibitor: Finasteride: Interfere with disease progression.
   b. α_1-adrenergic blocker: Prazosin/Terazosin/Tamsulosin: Provide symptomatic relief.
2. Surgical: Transurethral resection of prostate (TURP) is gold standard in the term of reduction of symptoms.

CHAPTER

6

Female Genital System

Leiomyoma of uterus

Description

It is a specimen of hemisection of uterus showing irregular nodular growths which are:
- Well-circumscribed
- Whitish in color
- Glistening surface
- Encircled by a fibrous capsule with a typical whorled appearance.
  Rest of the uterine muscle looks reddish brown.
  – So, the specimen is identified as "Leiomyoma of uterus" (Fig. 6.1).

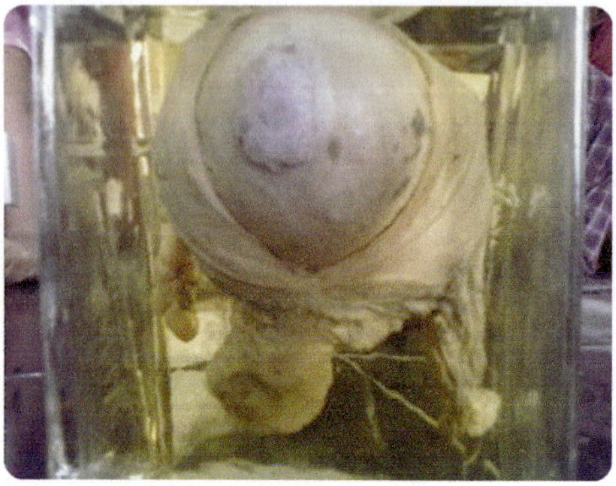

Fig. 6.1: Leiomyoma of uterus

What are the different types of uterine leiomyoma?

According to anatomical location it is classified as:
1. Intramural: Located within the body of uterus.
2. Submucus: When pushed towards uterine cavity.
3. Subserous: When pushed towards peritoneal cavity.

Describe the histology of leiomyoma.

- On microscopy, leiomyoma is composed of whorled bundles of smooth muscle cells that resemble the uninvolved myometrium (Fig. 6.2).

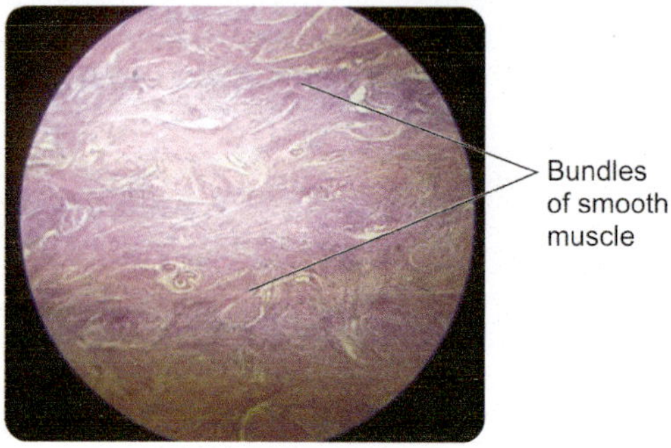

Fig. 6.2: Histology of leiomyoma

- Usually, the individual muscle cells are uniform in size and shape and have the characteristic oval nucleus and long bipolar cytoplasmic processes.

What is the cell of origin of leiomyoma?

Smooth muscle cell.

What is the malignant counterpart of leiomyoma?

Leiomyosarcoma.

What are the sites where leiomyoma are found?

The sites involved are (in decreased frequency):

1. Uterus (most common before the age of 40)
2. Cervix
3. Broad ligament
4. Ovary
5. Retroperitoneum
6. Skin
7. GIT, etc.

Theoretically, it may occur at any site in the body where there is a muscular vessel.

What is the minimum mitotic count for diagnosis of leiomyosarcoma?

10 per 10 high-power fields.

Carcinoma cervix

Description

It is a specimen of cervix and vaginal cuff showing an ulcerated growth with a rolled out margin.

- So, the specimen is identified as "Carcinoma cervix" (Figs 6.3A to C).

What are the different macroscopic types of carcinoma cervix?

1. Fungating type
2. Ulcerative type
3. Infiltrative type.

What are the main histological types of carcinoma cervix?

1. Squamous cell carcinoma (80%)
2. Adenocarcinoma (15%).

What is the causative agent of cervical carcinoma?

Human papilloma virus (HPV) type 16 and type 18.

What are the important risk factors for carcinoma cervix?

1. Age: Young woman of age: 25–45 years.
2. Past history of genital warts.
3. Marital status: Widowed/divorced/separated/multiple sexual partners.
4. Early marriage/early childbearing/repeated childbirth.
5. Continued use of oral contraceptive pills with high estrogen content.
6. Lower socioeconomic group: With poor genital hygiene.

Describe the main points of pathogenesis of cervical carcinoma by HPV.

- HPVs cannot infect the mature superficial squamous cells covering ectocervix/vagina/vulva.
- HPVs can only infect immature basal cells of the squamous epithelium in areas of epithelial breaks present at the squamocolumnar junction.
- The endocervix contains large areas of immature squamous metaplastic epithelium.
- So the endocervix is particularly vulnerable to HPV infection.
- After being integrated with the host genome; the HPV genome produces two viral proteins named E6 and

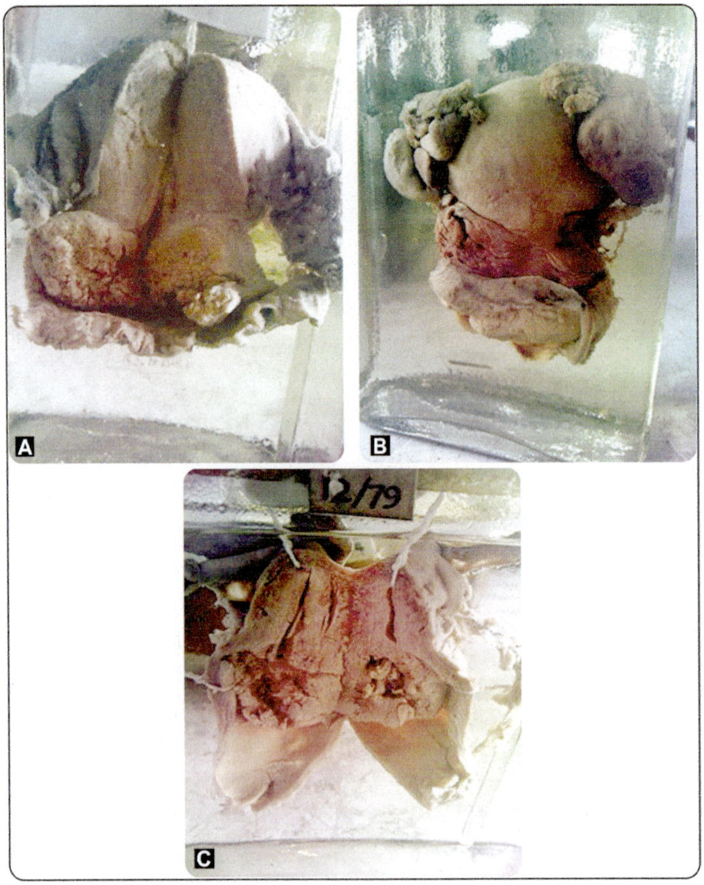

Figs 6.3A to C: Specimens of cervical carcinoma. A and B. Gross, and C. Cut section

E7, which are responsible primarily for the uncontrolled growth and differentiation of immature squamous epithelium of cervix. The mechanism how E6 and E7 work is as follows:

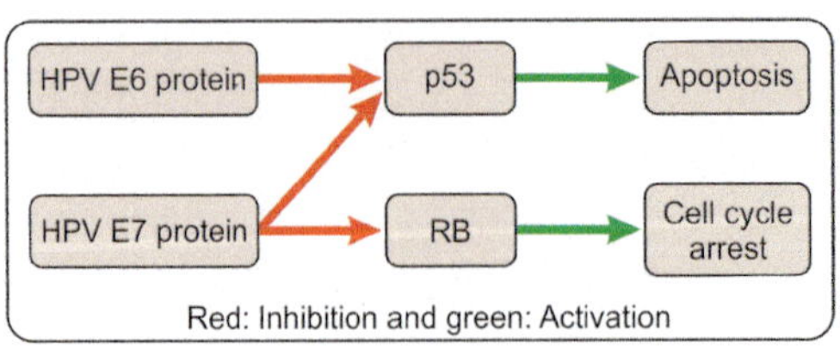

What is the natural course of events in the progression of cancer cervix?

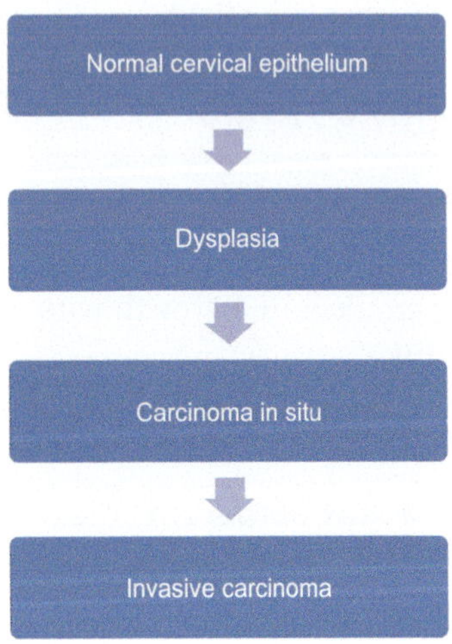

What is the classification system of cervical premalignant lesions?

Three different classification systems had been evolved to describe cervical premalignant lesions. They were based on:

1. Degree of dysplasia
2. Cervical intraepithelial neoplasia (CIN)
3. Squamous intraepithelial lesion (SIL): Most recent classification.
   - To understand the approach, all of these 3 systems are being discussed.

Dysplasia	CIN	SIL
Mild	CIN 1	LSIL*
Moderate	CIN 2	HSIL
Severe	CIN 3	HSIL
Carcinoma in situ	CIN 3	HSIL

*LSIL: Low grade SIL; HSIL: High grade SIL.

It should be mentioned that most of the LSIL does not progress to HSIL; but they eventually regress; so **LSIL is not regarded as a premalignant lesion**.

What do you mean by "Koilocytic atypia"? What is its importance?

- **Koilocyte**: It is defined as a squamous epithelial cell that has gone certain structural changes as a result of HPV infection.
- **Koilocytic atypia**: It is a cytopathic effect seen when HPV infects a squamous epithelial cell. It is characterized by:
  - Enlargement of the nucleus
  - Hyperchromasia (dark staining) of the nucleus
  - Irregular nuclear membrane
  - A clear area around the nucleus (Perinuclear halo) (Fig. 6.4).

Importance: The identification of "koilocytic atypia" in cervical microscopy is diagnostic of a dysplastic change within the cells. Now to classify the lesion into LSIL or HSIL, degree of epithelial thickness involvement is measured.

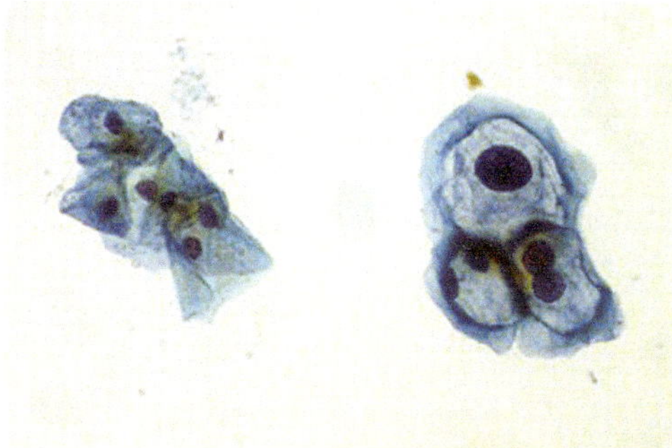

Fig. 6.4: Pap smear with groups of normal cervical cells on the left and HPV infected cells on the right; showing typical koilocytic changes:

- Enlarged nucleus
- Hyperchromasia
- Perineuclear halo.

(Courtesy of Dr Ed Uthman, MD)

How will you diagnose a cervical lesion as LSIL or HSIL?

Degree of SIL	Characteristic feature towards diagnosis
LSIL	The dysplastic immature squamous epithelial cells are confined to the lower 1/3rd of the total epithelial thickness
HSIL	The dysplastic immature squamous epithelial cells extend greater than lower 2/3rd of the total epithelial thickness

Name a marker that can detect dysplastic cervical epithelium.

Ki-67 (a marker of cellular proliferation).

How cervical carcinoma is staged?

Stages	Description
Stage 0	Carcinoma in situ (CIN III, HSIL); i.e. carcinoma is confined only to the surface layer of cervix
Stage 1	Carcinoma confined to the cervix
Stage 2	Carcinoma extends beyond the cervix but not to the pelvic wall. Carcinoma involves the vagina but not the lower-third

Contd...

Contd...

Stages	Description
Stage 3	Carcinoma has extended to the pelvic wall. The tumor involves the lower-third of the vagina
Stage 4	Carcinoma has extended beyond the true pelvis or has involved the mucosa of the bladder or rectum, also including metastatic dissemination

Name one test that is used for screening of carcinoma cervix?

1. Pap smear
2. Visual inspection with 5% acetic acid (VIA)
3. VIA with magnification (VIAM)
4. Visual inspection after application of Lugol's iodine (VILI).

What is the definitive treatment of carcinoma cervix?

Radical surgery and radiotherapy.

Dermoid cyst/benign cystic teratoma

Description

This is a specimen of enlarged ovary cut open to show a unilocular cyst (cyst having a single sac) containing sebum and hair follicles. It may also contain teeth or bone.

– So, the specimen is identified as "Benign cystic teratoma of ovary/ dermoid cyst" (Fig. 6.5).

What is a teratoma?

- Teratoma is an encapsulated tumor composed of tissues/organs which are foreign to the part in which it arises.
- It usually develops from all the 3 primitive germinal layers: Ectoderm, mesoderm and endoderm.

What is its origin?

Teratomas belong to a class called "Nonseminomatous germ cell tumors (NSGCT)". The tumors in the NSGCT group arise from 2 origins: Germ cells and embryonal cells. Teratomas are of germ cell origin.

What are the different sites where teratoma is found?

1. Gonads (the most common site)
2. Sacrococcygeal region
3. Retroperitoneum
4. Mediastinum

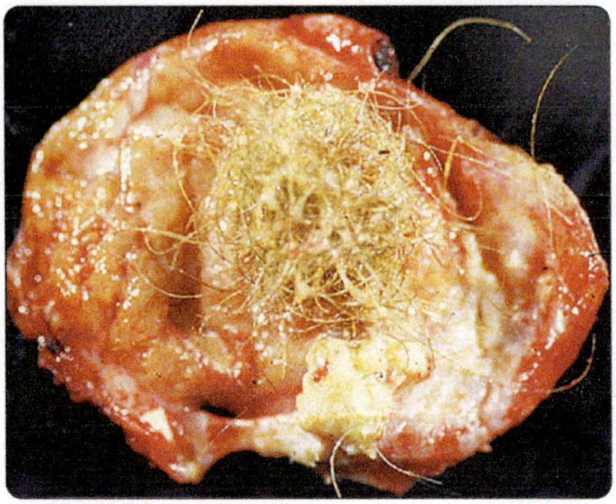

Fig. 6.5: Dermoid cyst/ Benign cystic teratoma. The cyst cavity is filled with a thick, greasy fluid and often contains cartilage, hair and well-formed teeth. Reproduced under the permission of "Health, Medicine and Anatomy Reference Pictures" (www.healthfavo.com)

5. Nasopharynx
6. Base of the skull, etc.

What are the different types of teratoma?

Teratoma is usually of 3 types:

1. Mature teratoma/benign cystic teratoma/dermoid cyst.
2. Immature teratoma/malignant teratoma.
3. Monodermal/specialized teratoma.

What are the characteristic features of a dermoid cyst?

1. Dermoid cyst usually contains hair and adnexal structures of the skin and other structures; which are derived from ectoderm (Fig. 6.6).
2. **As it contains only mature tissue, a dermoid cyst is benign as a rule**.
3. The wall of dermoid cyst is formed by stratified squamous epithelial cells, which very rarely may develop into squamous cell carcinoma in adults.
4. Infrequently, a dermoid cyst may contain tissues derived from all the 3 germ cell layers (Fig. 6.7).

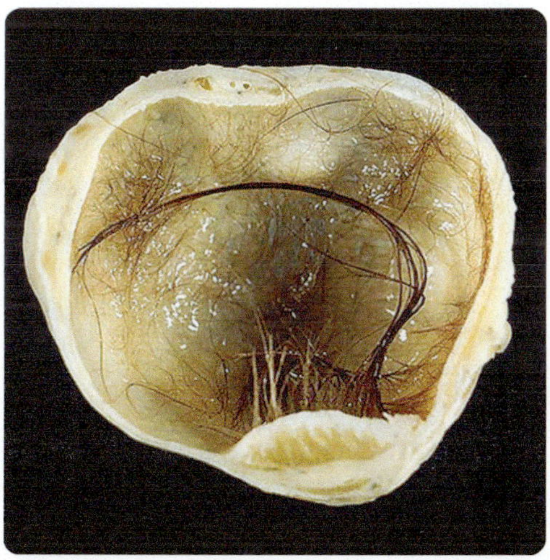

Fig. 6.6: Benign cystic teratoma of ovary showing abundant hair and other cutaneous structures. (Courtesy of Dr Ed Uthman, MD)

Describe the morphology of benign cystic teratoma.

- On histologic examination the cyst wall is composed of stratified squamous epithelium with:
  a. Sebaceous glands
  b. Hair shafts
  c. Skin, etc.
- In some cases structures from other germ layers can be identified, such as:
  a. Cartilage
  b. Bone
  c. Thyroid tissue
  d. Neural tissues.

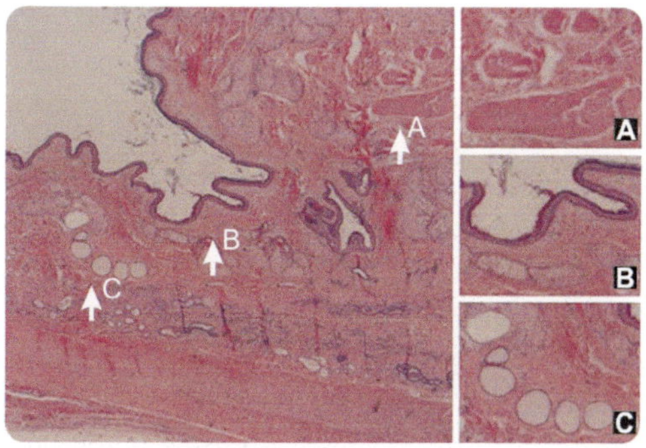

Fig. 6.7: Histology of a benign mature teratoma. A. Muscle, B. Skin and skin appendage, C. Mucous cyst. Reproduced under the permission of Korean Endocrine Journal and Dr Byung Joon Kim, Division of Endocrinology and Metabolism, Department of Internal Medicine, Konyang University College of Medicine, Korea

What are the complications of benign cystic teratoma?

1. Tortion of the cyst.
2. Rupture of the cyst with severe foreign body reaction in peritoneum.
3. Malignant transformation (in 1% of cases).

CHAPTER

7

Breast

Breast carcinoma

Description

- It is a specimen showing hemisection of breast with a grayish yellow growth.
- The growth is irregular in shape with poorly defined margins extending into the surrounding tissue.
- Nipple is retracted and skin on surface presents an orange peel like dimpled structure.
  - So, the specimen is identified as "Carcinoma breast" (Figs 7.1A and B).

(The growth, if felt, is hard and if cut, grating sound is heard).

Name some of the common genes which are mutated in breast carcinoma?

a. BRCA1
b. BRCA2
c. CHEK2
d. p53.
   - Mutations in these genes are associated with hereditary breast cancer.

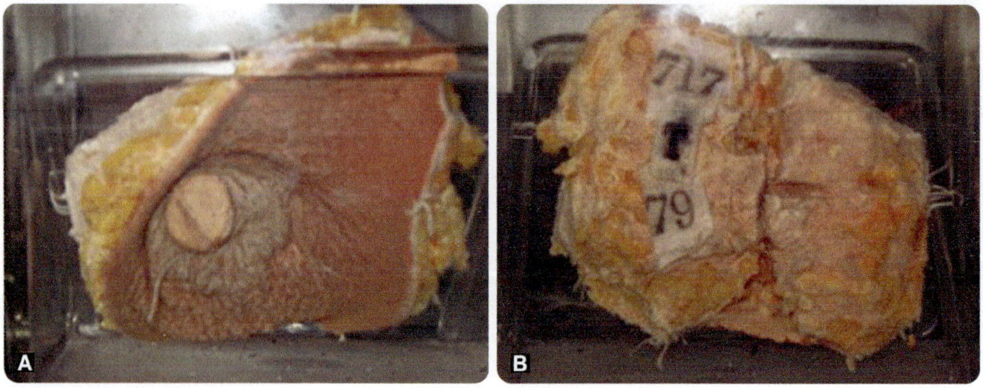

Figs 7.1A and B: Breast carcinoma

How will you classify carcinoma breast?

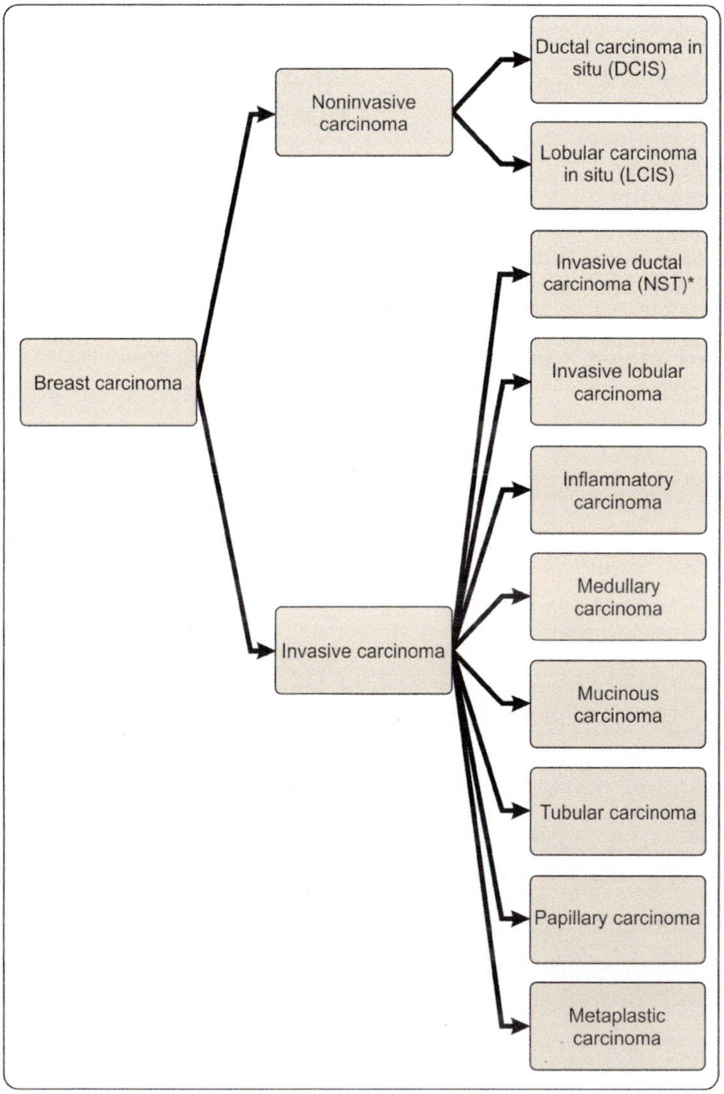

(*NST: No special type)

What are the proposed cells of origin of breast carcinoma?

- ER+ve breast carcinoma: Luminal cells.
- ER–ve breast carcinoma: Myoepithelial cells.

How will you diagnose a case of breast carcinoma?/ What is triple assessment?

If any patient presents with a breast lump/ other symptoms suspicious of carcinoma, the diagnosis should be made by a combination of:

1. Clinical assessment
2. Radiological study

3. Pathological examination with tissue sample.
   – It is called triple assessment.

- Triple assessment—

1. **Clinical assessment**:
   a. Age of the patient
   b. Clinical examination.
2. **Radiological study**:
   a. Mammography
   b. Ultrasound scan.
3. **Pathological examination**:
   a. FNAC: Fine needle aspiration cytology
   b. Breast core biopsy.

Which type of breast carcinoma has worst prognosis?

Inflammatory carcinoma.

Which type of breast carcinoma has most favorable prognosis?

Noninvasive carcinoma. Particularly LCIS.

What are the histological subtypes of DCIS?

1. Comedocarcinoma
2. Solid
3. Cribriform
4. Papillary
5. Micropapillary.

What are the gene expression profiles of various types of invasive ductal carcinoma/ NST?

Type of invasive ductal carcinoma	*ER (Estrogen receptor)*	*PR (Progesterone receptor)*	*HER2/neu*	*Comment*
Luminal A	+	+	–	Most common invasive ductal carcinoma
Luminal B	+	+	+	Triple positive phenotype
Basal-like	–	–	–	Triple negative phenotype
Normal breast-like	+	+	–	Morphology similar to normal breast tissue
HER2 positive	–	–	+	Treated with Herceptin (monoclonal antibody against HER2/ neu)

What are the different modes of metastasis of breast carcinoma?

Route of spread	*Site of metastasis*
Lymphatic	• Axillary lymph node • Internal mammary node • Mediastinal lymph node • Supraclavicular lymph node • Lymphatic spread may extend to the contralateral breast
Hematogenous	• Lung • Liver • Bones • Adrenal • Brain • Ovary
Transcelomic spread	Spread to ovary forming Krukenberg's tumor

How will you stage breast cancer?

Stages	*Subdivision*	*Extent [T]*	*Positive lymph nodes [N]*	*Metastasis [M]*
0		DCIS/ LCIS	0	–
1		Invasive CA ≤ 2cm	0	–
2	2A 2B	Invasive CA >2 cm Invasive CA <5 cm	0 1–3	– –
3	3A 3B 3C	Invasive CA >5 cm Any size invasive CA Invasive CA with skin or chest wall involvement or inflammatory carcinoma	1–3 ≥4 –Ve/ +Ve	– – –
4		Any size invasive CA	–Ve/ +Ve	+

Give the name of one benign, one intermediate and one malignant tumors of breast.

1. Benign: Fibroadenoma
2. Intermediate: Phyllodes tumor
3. Malignant: Invasive ductal carcinoma.

CHAPTER

8

Bones and Joints

Sequestrum

Description

It is a specimen of white, dry, irregular ring-shaped piece of bone with granular surface.

- So, this is a specimen of "Ring sequestrum" (Figs 8.1A and B).

What is a sequestrum?

It is a piece of necrosed bone which gets separated from living tissue in case of chronic osteomyelitis.

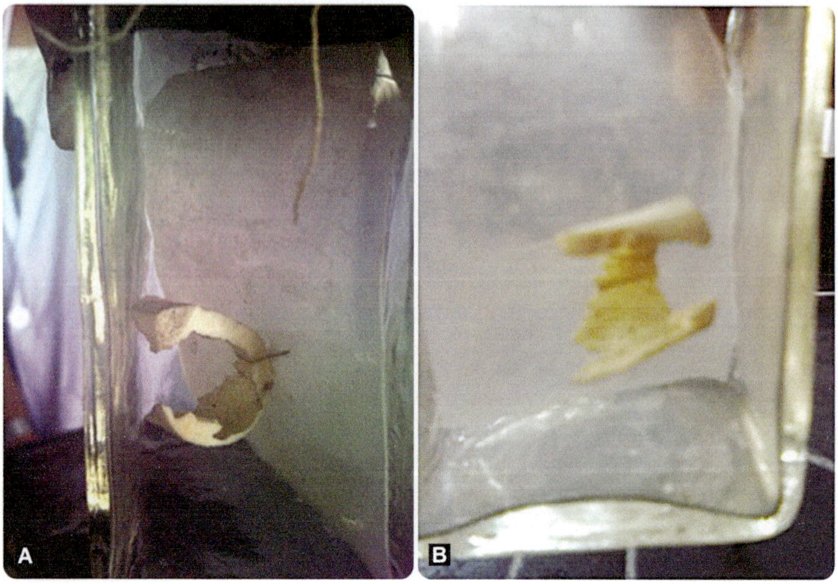

Figs 8.1A and B: Sequestrum

What is involucrum?

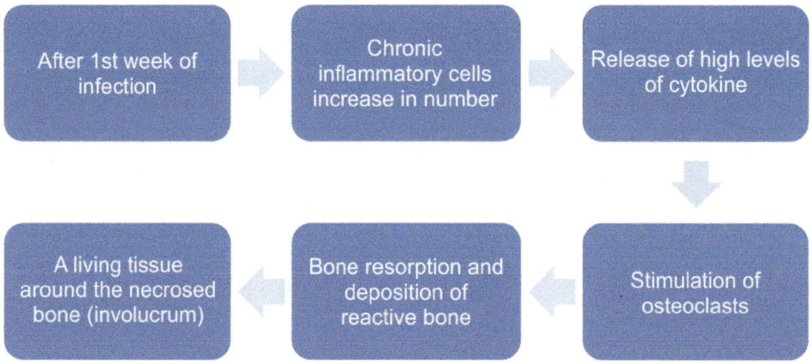

- After the above sequence of events in chronic osteomyelitis, when the newly deposited bone forms a piece of living tissue around the segment of devitalized infected bone, it is known as an involucrum.

What are the main causative agents of pyogenic osteomyelitis?

1. *Staphylococcus aureus* (80–90% of cases: more common in intravenous drug abusers).
2. *Escherichia coli,* Pseudomonas, and Klebsiella (individuals with genitourinary tract infections).
3. Mixed bacterial infections (inoculation of organisms during surgery or open fractures).
4. *Haemophilus influenzae* (neonatal period).
5. Salmonella (sickle cell disease).
6. In almost 50% of cases, no organisms can be isolated.

What is the most common organism responsible for osteomyelitis?

Staphylococcus aureus.

How the organisms lodge into the bone and where?

- Metaphysis of long bone is a highly vascularized zone, where the medullary arteries and medullary veins branch into capillaries in a specific pattern called "Hairpin arrangement" (Fig. 8.2).
- The blood stasis resulting from such an arrangement is responsible for the metaphysis being a favorable site for bacteria to settle.
- So the organisms pass through the bone, get lodged in the metaphysis.
- Lower femoral metaphysis is the most common site.

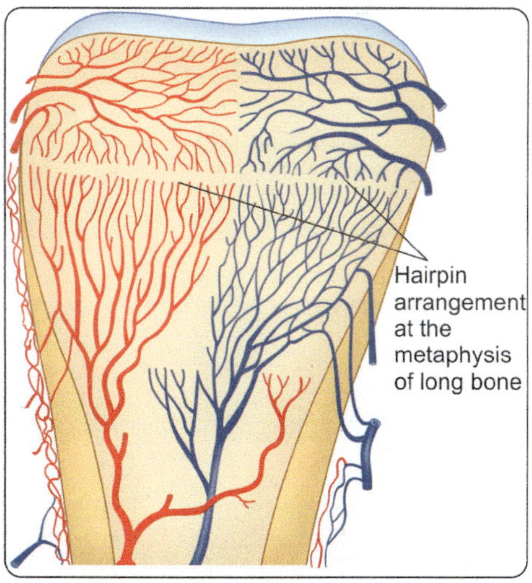

Fig. 8.2: Hairpin arrangement of medullary veins and arteries

How will you diagnose a case of acute and chronic osteomyelitis?

Parameters	*Acute osteomyelitis*	*Chronic osteomyelitis*
Presenting complaint	Acute onset of pain and swelling at the end of a bone, associated with systemic features of infection like fever	A chronic discharging sinus is the most common presenting complaint. They may heal for short periods; only to reappear with each acute exacerbation
Examination findings	The patient is febrile and dehydrated with classical signs of inflammation: redness/heat, etc. localized to the metaphysis of the bone	A chronic discharging sinus with a thickened bone and mild tenderness on deep palpation; adjacent joint may be stiff due to extensive scarring of soft tissues
Blood	PMN (polymorphonuclear) leukocytosis with an elevated ESR	Normal
X-ray	Periosteal new bone deposition at the metaphysis	– Thickening of cortex – Focal areas of sclerosis – Sequestrum (dead piece of bone) surrounded by granulation tissue – Involucrum (dense sclerotic lesion overlying the sequestrum) may be seen

Describe the pathogenesis of pyogenic osteomyelitis in short.

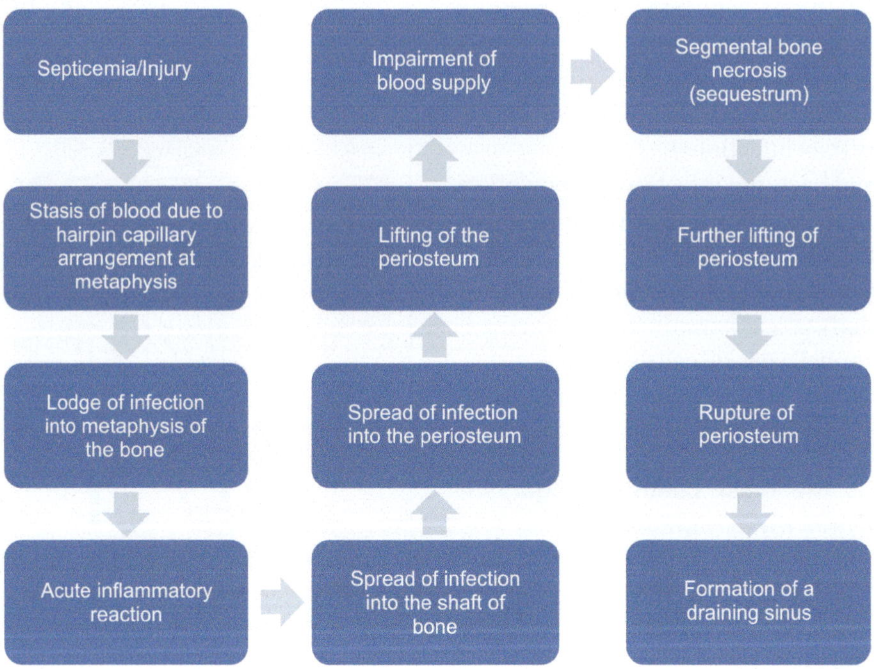

- After the first week the number of chronic inflammatory cells increases and their release of cytokines stimulate osteoclastic bone resorption and at the same time, deposition of reactive bone in the periphery.
- When the newly deposited bone forms a piece of living tissue around the necrosed bone segment, it is known as an involucrum.

What are the complications of acute and chronic osteomyelitis?

Complications of acute osteomyelitis	*Complications of chronic osteomyelitis*
Chronic osteomyelitis (most commonly due to a delay in diagnosis)	Episodes of acute exacerbation (due to reactivation of infection)
Acute pyogenic arthritis (occurs in case of an intra-articular joint, e.g. hip)	Growth abnormalities: • Shortening • Lengthening • Deformities
Pathological fractures	Pathological fractures
Growth plate disturbances	Joint stiffness
Sinus tract malignancy	Amyloidosis

Tuberculosis of spine (Pott's disease)

Description

This is a specimen of hemisection of a spine showing destruction of a part of vertebra and intervertebral disc.

- So, the specimen is identified as "Tuberculosis of spine/Pott's disease" (Figs 8.3A and B).

Why this is not a metastatic lesion?

This is not a metastatic lesion because in the metastatic lesion, intervertebral discs are not affected.

Which are the most common sites of involvement of tuberculous osteomyelitis?

1. Spine (especially lumbar and thoracic vertebrae)
2. Knee
3. Hip.

What is the incidence of a pulmonary TB patient to have an osseous infection?

1–3 %.

Why "Night crying" is characteristic of Pott's disease?

1. The affected portions of spine are supported while awake (in the day time) by muscular spasm.
2. But in the time of sleeping (at night), muscles relax which allows painful movements to take place. This intense pain is responsible for the night cries in children.

What are the complications of TB spine?

1. Severe destruction of vertebrae→ Permanent compression fractures → Deformities (scoliosis/ kyphosis)
2. Compression of the spinal cord → Neurologic deficits
3. Tuberculous arthritis
4. Sinus tract formation
5. Psoas abscess
6. Amyloidosis.

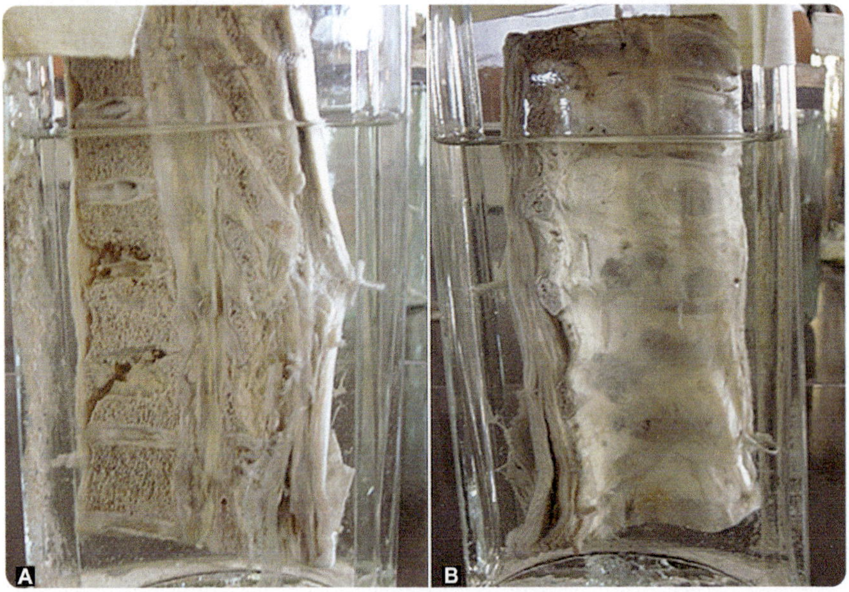

Figs 8.3A and B: Tuberculosis of spine. A. Front view and B. Back view

Giant cell tumor of bone

Description

- It is a specimen showing a fusiform growth at the end of ulna.
- The growth has expanded from inner portion of the bone, pressing the cortical bone into a thin shell at the surface of the growth.
- Cut surface is dark tan in color.
- Blackish areas of hemorrhage, necrosis and cystic change are being seen.
  - So, the specimen is identified as "Giant cell tumor of bone/osteoclastoma" (Figs 8.4A and B).

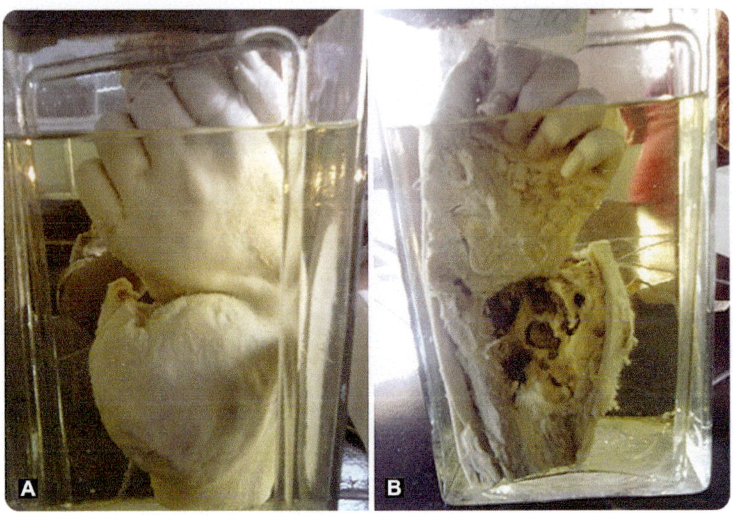

Figs 8.4A and B: Giant cell tumors (GCT) of bone

What is the most common site of a GCT bone?

Around the knee joint. (Then comes the distal radius and sacrum).

Which part of the bone is commonly affected?

- **Adult**: Metaphysis and epiphysis.
- **Adolescent**: Metaphysis.

What is the behavior of giant cell tumor of bone?

GCT of bone is a benign but locally aggressive tumor.

Describe the morphological features of a GCT.

- The tumor stroma is highly vascular.
- They are mostly composed of uniform oval mononuclear cells that represent the proliferating component of the tumor.
- There are numerous osteoclast-type giant cells having ≥100 nuclei scattered within this background; giving the name "Osteoclastoma" (Fig. 8.5).
- Necrosis and hemorrhage are commonly seen.

What is the cell of origin of GCT?

GCT bone is thought to be of mesenchymal origin.

What are the criteria of malignancy in a GCT of bone?

1. Pleomorphism
2. Increased mitosis of stromal cells
3. Reduction in the number and size of giant cells.

How will you diagnose a case of GCT?

Confirmation of the diagnosis: We will take an anteroposterior view and a lateral view X-ray of the affected joint. The following characteristic features will help us differentiating it from other solitary lytic lesions of the bone.

Positive points:

A. Occurs only with a closed growth plate.
B. Eccentric location of the tumor.
C. Well-defined with nonsclerotic margins.

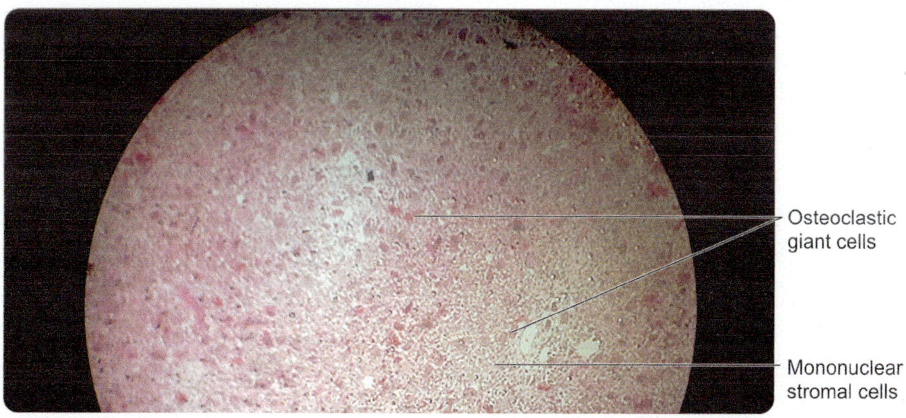

Fig. 8.5: Light microscopy of giant cell tumor illustrating an abundance of multinucleated giant cells with a background of mononuclear stromal cells

D. The characteristic "Soap bubble appearance", i.e. the trabeculae of the remaining bone traversing the tumor, giving the tumor a "Sac-like appearance" (Fig. 8.6).

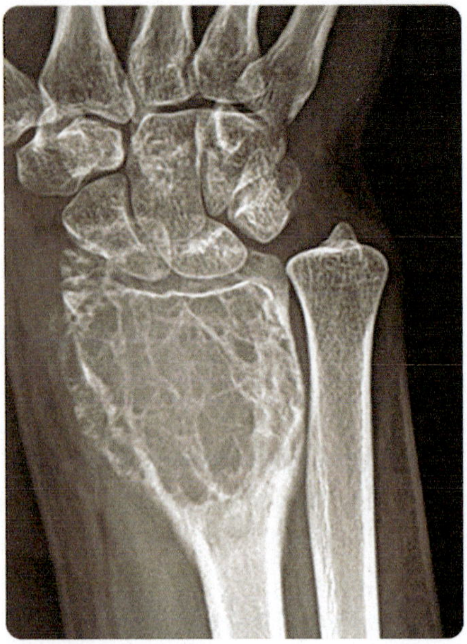

Fig. 8.6: GCT of distal radius
Note: The subarticular location, expansile nature and characteristic "Soap bubble appearance."(Reproduced under the permission of Dr Wael Nemattalla, Radiopaedia.org)

Negative points:

A. No calcification and no new bone formation within the tumor.
B. The tumor usually does not invade the adjacent joint(s).

Name some of the common bone lesions which contain osteoclastic giant cells.

1. Giant cell tumor of bone
2. Simple bone cyst
3. Aneurysmal bone cyst
4. Chondromyxoid fibroma
5. Benign chondroblastoma
6. Brown tumor of hyperparathyroidism.

Osteosarcoma

Description

- It is a specimen of a long bone showing bulky gray-white growth at the end of the bone.
- Cut surface is grayish white with areas of hemorrhage and necrosis.
- The bone cortex is destroyed.
  - So, the specimen is identified as "Osteosarcoma" (Fig. 8.7).

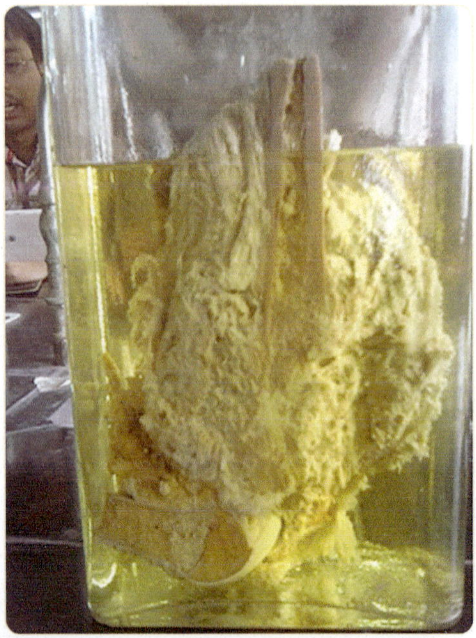

Fig. 8.7: Osteosarcoma

What is the cell of origin?

Primitive mesenchymal cell.

What are the types of osteosarcoma?

There are two types of osteosarcoma:

1. **Primary osteosarcoma**:
   I. It is usually seen in 15–25 years of age group.
   II. It occurs without any past history of known premalignant conditions of bone but it is much more malignant than the secondary osteosarcoma.

2. **Secondary osteosarcoma**:
   I. It is usually seen in >45 years of age.
   II. It occurs with a past history of known premalignant conditions of bone (like Paget's disease, fibrous dysplasia of bone, irradiation to bones, multiple osteochondroma, etc.).

What are the different histological types of osteosarcoma?

A. **Osteoblastic type**: With extensive new bone formation.
B. **Chondroid type**: With basic cell being a cartilage cell.
C. **Fibroblastic type**: With basic cell being a fibroblast.
D. **Osteolytic type**: A predominantly lytic tumor.

What are the bones/joints commonly involved in osteosarcoma?

1. Knee joint (most common)
2. Hip joint
3. Shoulder joint.

What is the most common type of osteosarcoma?

The most common subtype arises in the metaphysis of long bones and is primary, solitary, intramedullary, and poorly differentiated in nature.

Describe the invasion of long bones by osteosarcoma.

- They spread extensively in the medullary canal, infiltrating and replacing the marrow.
- When joint invasion occurs, the tumor grows into it in either of the 2 ways:
1. Along the muscle tendons
2. Along the attachment site of the joint capsule.
- The tumors frequently destroy the surrounding cortices and produce soft tissue abscesses.

Describe the morphology of osteosarcoma.

- The formation of bone by the tumor cells is characteristic of osteosarcoma.
- The neoplastic bone forms in a characteristic dense, lace-like pattern (Fig. 8.8).
- The tumor cells frequently have large hyperchromatic nuclei.
- Tumor giant cells are commonly seen.

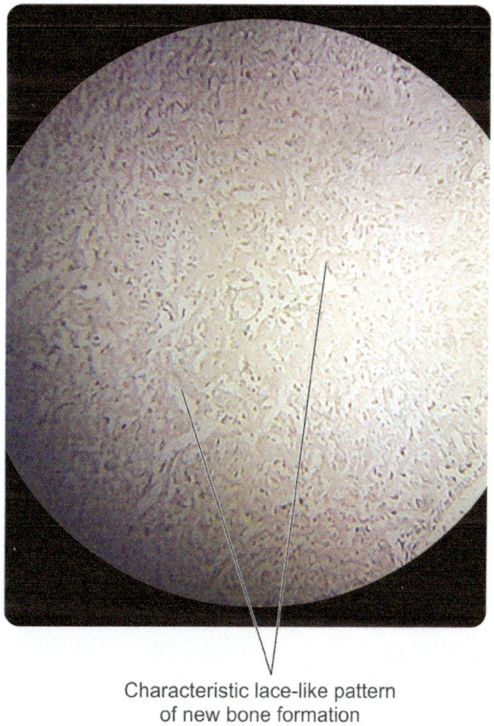

Fig. 8.8: Morphology of osteosarcoma

Is the tumor aggressive? If yes, how will you detect its aggressiveness?

Yes, the tumor appears to be aggressive, metastasizing frequently all over the body, at first to the lung.

To detect the aggressiveness/metastasis of the tumor, a SAP (serum alkaline phosphates test) has to be done.

Although it is a nonspecific test, but a *higher value after initial lowering* after tumor excision indicates new metastasis of residual tumor/recurrence.

How will you confirm a diagnosis of osteosarcoma?

A. **X-ray**:
   I. An area of irregular destruction of metaphysis.
   II. The cortex is eroded.
   III. There is new bone formation in the matrix of the tumor, which lifts the periosteum.
   IV. A triangular area of subperiosteal new bone is seen in the tumor-cortex junction; known as "Codman's triangle" (Fig. 8.9).
   V. New bone is laid down along the blood vessels growing centrifugally within the tumor; responsible for a "Sunray appearance".

B. **Open biopsy**:

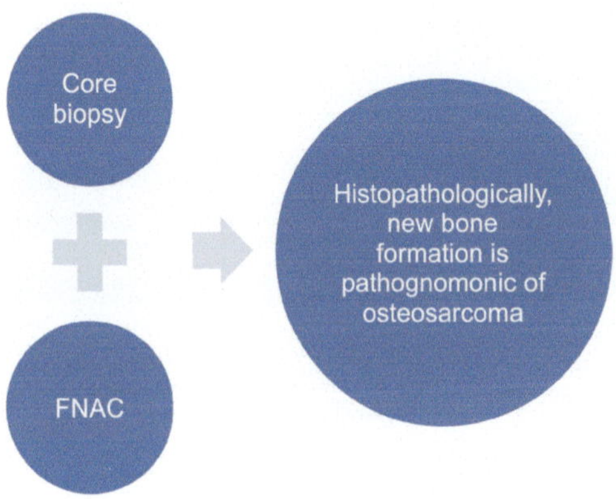

What is Codman's triangle? Name some cases where it is seen.

It is a triangular area of new subperiosteal bone formation usually formed when a tumor/lesion of the bone lifts the periosteum away from the bone.

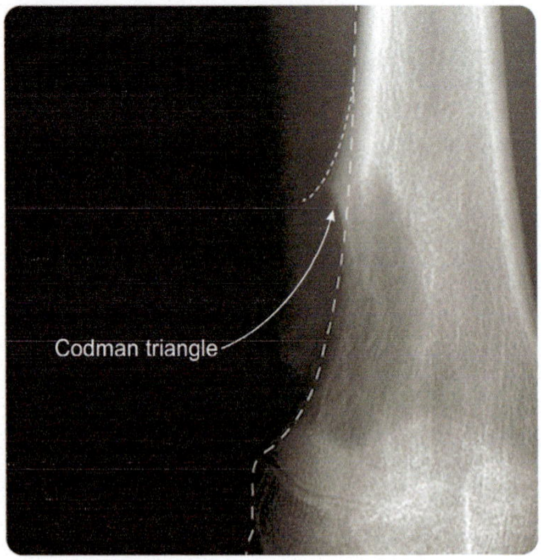

Fig. 8.9: Codman's triangle. Courtesy of Dr frask Gaillard and Radiopaedia.org.

Main causes for Codman's triangle:
- Osteosarcoma
- Ewing's sarcoma
- Subperiosteal abscess.

Name some other osteoblastic tumors of bone.

1. Osteoma
2. Osteoid sarcoma
3. Osteoblastoma
4. Osteochondroma.

CHAPTER 9

Respiratory System

At first we will recapitulate the basic gross anatomy of lung (Fig. 9.1).

Lobar pneumonia of lung

Description

- The specimen is a cut section of lung showing solidification of a lobe.
- The area of solidification looks solid and yellowish gray in color.
  - So, the specimen is identified as "Lobar pneumonia of lung" (Fig. 9.2).

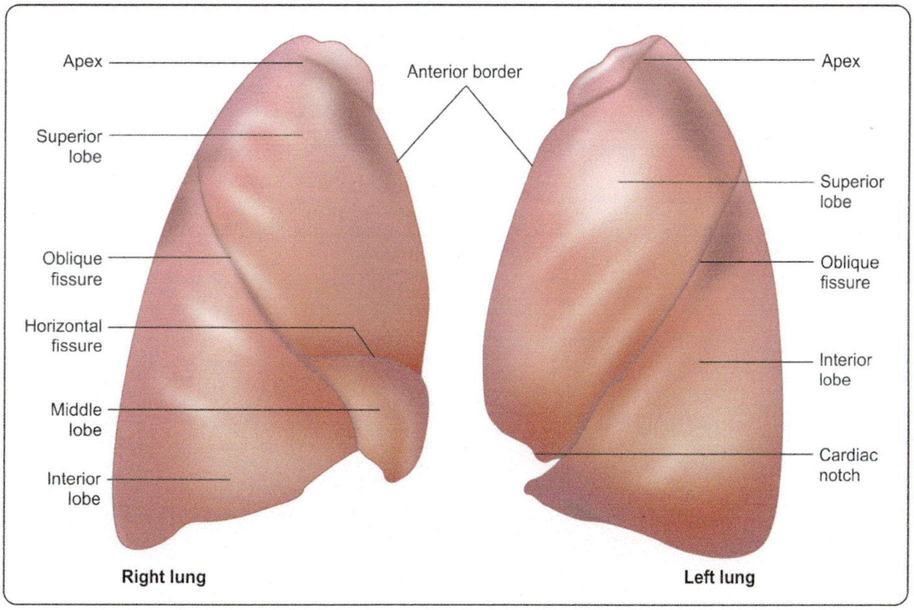

Fig. 9.1: Basic anatomy of lung

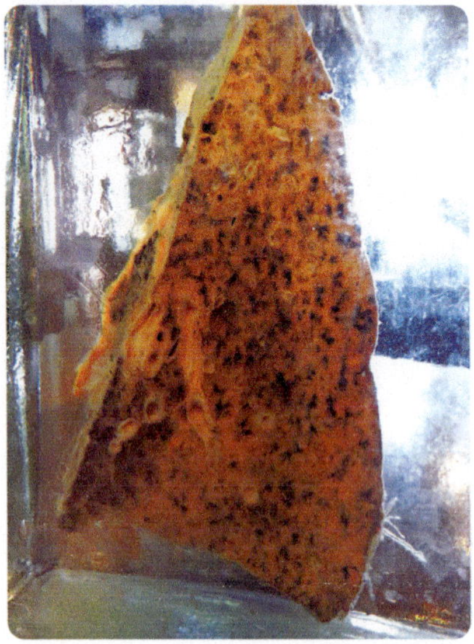

Fig. 9.2: Lobar pneumonia of lung. Cut surface of lung showing gray-white consolidated areas, dry, granular in appearance with liver like consistency

What are the causative agents of lobar pneumonia of lung?

Types of pneumonia	Causative agents
Community-acquired acute pneumonia	1. *Streptococcus pneumoniae* 2. *Haemophilus influenzae* 3. *Moraxella catarrhalis* 4. *Staphylococcus aureus* 5. *Legionella pneumophila* 6. *Klebsiella pneumoniae* 7. Pseudomonas spp
Community-acquired atypical pneumonia	1. *Mycoplasma pneumoniae* 2. Chlamydia spp. (*C. pneumoniae, C. psittaci, C. trachomatis*) 3. Coxiella burnetii (Q fever) 4. Viruses: A. Influenza A and B (adults) B. Parainfluenza virus (children) C. Adenovirus D. Respiratory syncytial virus E. SARS virus
Hospital-acquired pneumonia	1. *Klebsiella pneumoniae* 2. *Escherichia coli* 3. Pseudomonas spp 4. *Staphylococcus aureus* (usually penicillin resistant)

What is meant by consolidation?

Replacement of alveolar air by inflammatory infiltrates.

Why is this not a specimen of bronchopneumonia?

This is not a specimen of bronchopneumonia because bronchopneumonia is patchy in distribution and usually does not involve the whole lobe (Fig. 9.3).

What are the histological stages in lobar pneumonia?

1. Stage of congestion
2. Stage of red hepatization
3. Stage of gray hepatization
4. Stage of resolution.

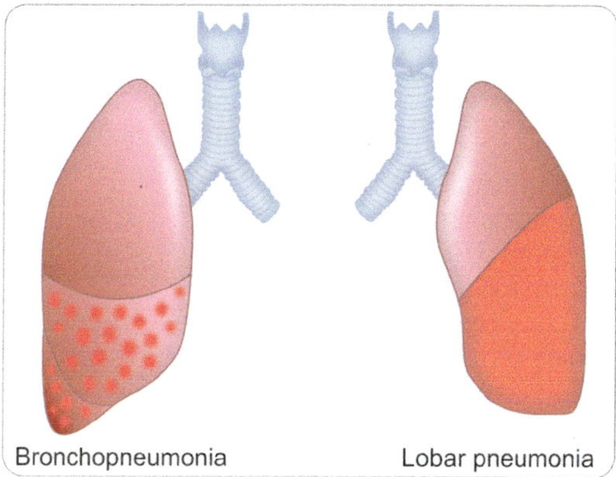

Fig. 9.3: Bronchopneumonia and lobar pneumonia of lung

Describe the stages of lobar pneumonia in short.

Stages of	*Duration*	*Gross appearance*	*Microscopic appearance*
Congestion	1–2 days	Affected lung is: • Enlarged • Heavy • Congested • Dark red in color	Typical features of acute inflammation: • Dilation and congestion of capillaries • Eosinophilic edema fluid in the air spaces • Numerous bacteria in the alveolar fluid
Red hepatization	2–4 days	Cut surface reveals: • Granularity • Red pink in color • Firm with liver-like consistency	• The eosinophilic edema fluid is replaced by fibrin strands • Marked neutrophilic exudate with extravasation of RBCs is seen
Gray hepatization	4–8 days	Cut surface reveals: • Granularity • Gray in color • Firm with liver-like consistency	• Fibrin strands are denser • Neutrophils and RBC reduce in number • Organisms are less numerous
Resolution	8th day to next 1–3 weeks	Affected lobe is gradually restored due to liquefaction of fibrin strands by enzymatic action	• Macrophages are the dominant cells • Alveolar capillaries are engorged • Progressive removal of cellular exudate • Restoration of normal lung parenchyma (with aeration)

What are the complications associated with lobar pneumonia?

1. Empyema
2. Lung abscess
3. Septicemia
4. Delayed resolution
5. Organization and fibrosis.

Miliary tuberculosis of lung

Description

It is a specimen of a longitudinal section of lung showing numerous uniform small millet size white spots (tubercles) surrounded by areas of intense congestion.

- So, the specimen is identified as "Miliary tuberculosis of lung" (Figs 9.4A and B).

What does the term "Miliary" suggest?

The adjective "miliary" is derived from the similarity of the foci of consolidations to millet seeds.

How does one get Miliary TB of lung?

- Miliary pulmonary disease is sequelae of progressive TB.
- It occurs when organisms (tubercle bacilli) draining through lymphatics enter the venous blood and circulate back to the lung.

What are the usual histological findings?

- Individual lesions are either microscopic or small (2 mm) visible foci of yellow-white consolidation scattered throughout the lung parenchyma.
- Miliary lesions may expand and coalesce, resulting in consolidation of large regions or even whole lobes of the lung.

Fibrocaseous tuberculosis of lung

Description

- It is a specimen of lung showing some thick-walled cavities lined by yellowish-gray caseous material.
- The walls of the cavities are fibrotic and smooth.
- Bronchi and blood vessels are showing thickening.
  - So, the specimen is diagnosed as "Fibrocaseous tuberculosis of lung" (Fig. 9.5).

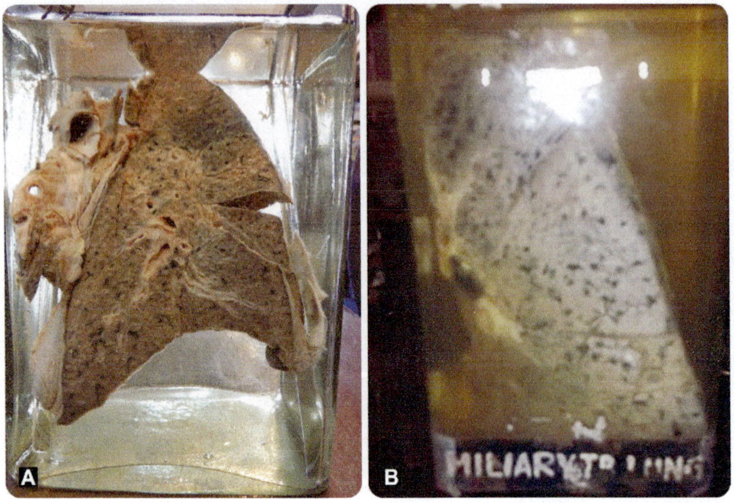

Figs 9.4A and B: Miliary tuberculosis of lung (Courtesy: Rajkumar Elanjeran, Gandhi Medical College, Hyderabad)

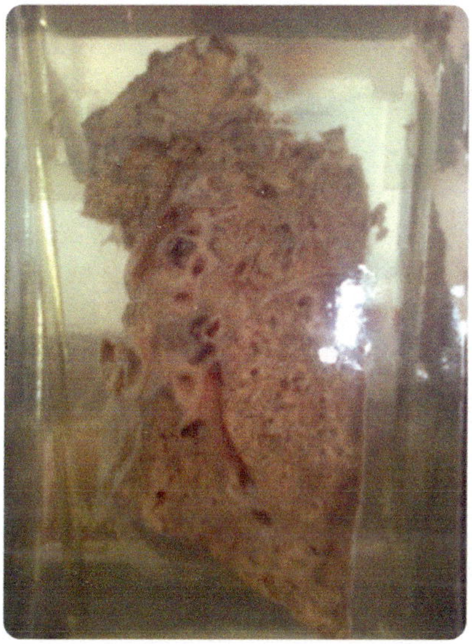

Fig. 9.5: Fibrocaseous tuberculosis of lung

Tuberculosis

What are the forms of tuberculosis in the lung?

a. Primary TB
b. Secondary TB
c. Progressive TB
d. Miliary TB.

What is Ghon's focus?

- Typically, the inhaled tubercle bacilli implant just above/just below the interlobar fissure (between the upper and lower lobes) and beneath the pleural membrane (so-called subpleural lesion).
- As sensitization develops, a 1–1.5 cm area of gray-white inflammation with consolidation emerges, known as the Ghon's focus.
- In most cases, the center of this focus undergoes caseous necrosis.

What is Ghon's complex?

- In primary TB of lung, tubercle bacilli (in free or phagocytosed form) drain to the regional lymph nodes, which often caseate.
- Ghon's complex is the initial lesion of primary TB. It consists of:
  A. A subpleural lesion, just above/ just below the interlobar fissure (between upper and lower lobes)
  B. Enlarged caseous peribronchial lymph nodes.

What is the fate of Ghon complex?

- It heals in about 90% of cases by:
  - Fibrosis
  - Calcification
  - Ossification.
- In unfavorable cases (10%), increased hypersensitivity reaction leads to progressive pulmonary TB.

When does secondary TB occur?

- Secondary tuberculosis is the pattern of disease that arises in a previously sensitized host.
- It commonly appears many years after the initial infection, usually when host resistance is weakened.
- It most commonly stems from reactivation of a latent infection.

What is Assman's focus?

- In secondary TB, the initial lesion is seen characteristically at the apex of the upper lobe of a lung (so-called apical lesion).
- Usually there is only little lymph node involvement (usually infraclavicular lymph node).
- This initial apical lesion in secondary TB (consisting of apical lesion and infraclavicular lymph node involvement) is called Assman's focus.
- Histologically, similar to Ghon focus, it has a central caseous necrosis which is surrounded by a granulomatous inflammatory reaction.
- In most cases, destruction of lung tissues leads to cavitation.

Describe the lesions found in progressive pulmonary TB.

- Progressive pulmonary TB may be a

consequence of progression of both primary and secondary TB.

- In a typical case, the initial lesion (subpleural lesion and apical lesion in primary and secondary TB, respectively) enlarges and erodes into the adjacent lung tissue and finally, into a bronchus.
- Through the eroded bronchus, the partially liquefied caseous necrotic tissue is drained, leaving a ragged, irregular cavity; the walls of the cavity become fibrotic.
- Growth and multiplication of tubercle bacilli are extensively enhanced in this condition as a cavity provides increased oxygen tension.
- This stage of the disease is called "Fibrocaseous TB of lung".
- If disease is not treated at this point, it may progress to involve the entire lobe with marked tissue destruction and fibrosis; resulting in "Tuberculous bronchopneumonia".
- When organisms draining through the lymphatics enter venous blood and circulate back to the lung, it results in "Miliary tuberculosis", small foci of consolidation spread throughout the lung, resulting in large areas of consolidation when they coalesce.

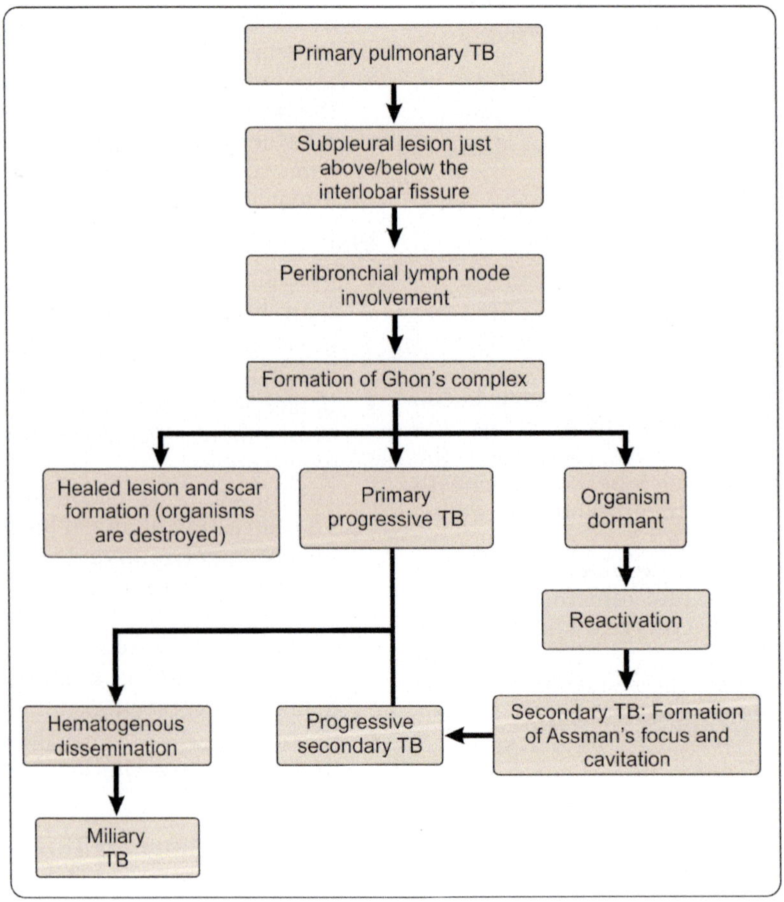

What is isolated tuberculosis?

- It may appear in any of the organs or tissues where the tubercle bacilli lodge hematogenously.
- Organs that are commonly involved include:
  1. The meninges (tuberculous meningitis)
  2. Kidneys (renal tuberculosis)
  3. Adrenals (formerly an important cause of addison disease)
  4. Bones (osteomyelitis)
  5. Fallopian tubes (salpingitis)
  6. Vertebrae (pott disease).

What is the most common presenting feature of extrapulmonary TB?

- Lymphadenitis is the most frequent presentation of extrapulmonary tuberculosis, usually occurring in the cervical region (scrofula).
- In HIV-negative individuals, lymphadenitis tends to be unifocal and localized.
- HIV-positive people almost always have multifocal disease and systemic symptoms.

What is nonreactive TB?

- In cases of very low host resistance (as in old age, AIDS, leukemia, persons receiving immunosuppressive drugs, etc.), the lesions show no cellular response.
- The lesions contain high amount of tubercle bacilli and are highly infective.

What is the confirmatory diagnosis of tuberculosis?

- Culture is the gold standard because it also allows testing of drug susceptibility.
- Conventional cultures require upto 10 weeks, but culture in liquid media can provide the result within 2 weeks.

What is the hallmark of activity and immunity in chronic TB infection?

Caseation and fibrosis, respectively.

Describe the histology of a tubercle.

- Section showing histology of lymph node.
- There is an area of granuloma containing: (Fig. 9.6)
  - Central necrosis with amorphous granular debris surrounded by focus of activated macrophages (epithelioid cells), rimmed by fibroblasts, lymphocytes, histiocytes, occasional Langhans giant cells.
  - It also may contain variable numbers of acid-fast bacilli.

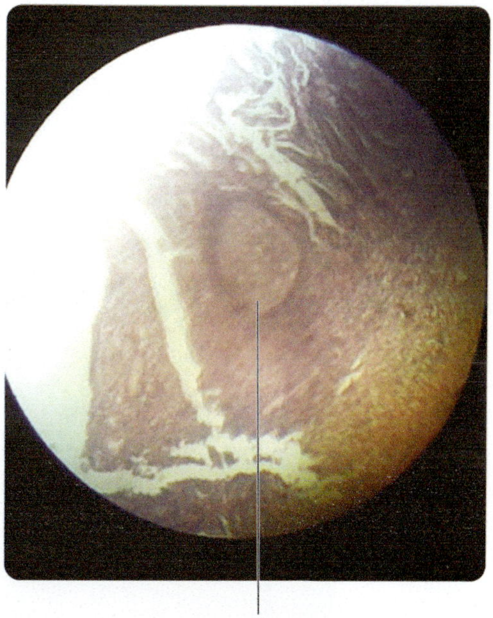

Fig. 9.6: Slide showing granuloma in a case of intestinal TB

Bronchogenic carcinoma

Description

- It is a specimen of lung exposing main and major bronchi.
- There is a yellowish-white and darkish growth arising from major bronchus, spreading both within and outside the bronchus and in the wall.
  - So, the specimen is identified as "Bronchogenic carcinoma" (Figs 9.7A and B).

What are the predisposing factors to CA lung?

1. Cigaret smoking: Most important single risk factor.
2. Industrial hazards:
   - High dose ionizing radiation
   - Asbestos
   - Uranium
   - Nickel
   - Chromium.
3. Air pollution:
   - Radon.
4. Genetic susceptibility: Mutations in the following genes are commonly associated with lung cancer:
   - c-MYC
   - KRAS
   - EGFR
   - c-MET
   - c-KIT
   - CYP1A1.

Describe the histologic classification of bronchogenic carcinoma.

1. Squamous cell carcinoma
2. Small-cell carcinoma
3. Adenocarcinoma:
   a. Acinar
   b. Papillary
   c. Bronchioloalveolar
   d. Solid
   e. Mixed subtypes.
4. Large-cell carcinoma.
5. Adenosquamous carcinoma.
6. Carcinoid tumor:
   a. Typical
   b. Atypical
7. Carcinomas of salivary gland type.

From which area does lung carcinoma originate?

- Lung carcinomas arise most often in and about the *hilus of the lung*.
- About 75% of the lesions take their origin from first-order, second-order, and third-order bronchi.
- Some of the primary carcinomas of the lung arise in the periphery of the lung from the alveolar septal cells or terminal bronchioles.

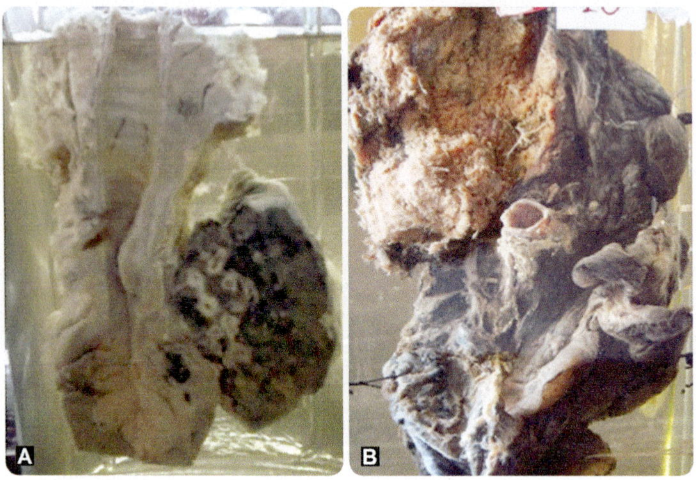

Figs 9.7A and B: Bronchogenic carcinoma

Describe how lung carcinoma destroys lung tissue and additional structures.

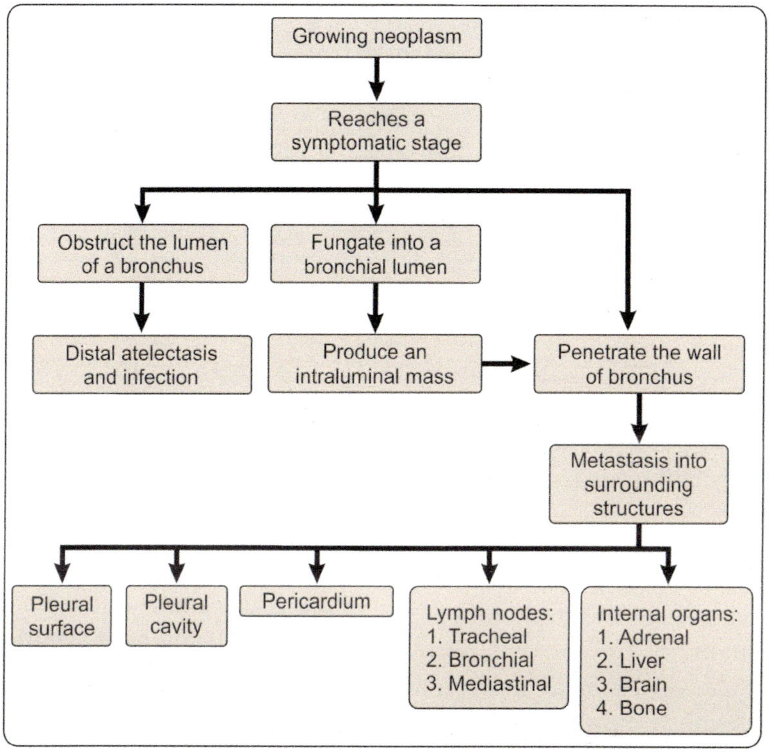

Describe the path of metastasis of lung carcinoma.

- Distant spread of lung carcinoma occurs through both lymphatic and hematogenous pathways.
- These tumors often spread early throughout the body except for squamous cell carcinoma, which metastasizes outside the thorax late.
- The **adrenals** are most commonly involved in >50% of cases.
- The liver, brain and bone are also favorable sites of metastases.

What is the specialty of growth pattern of bronchioloalveolar carcinoma?

- This type of carcinoma arises in the terminal bronchioloalveolar regions.
- Histologically, the tumor is characterized by a pure bronchioloalveolar growth pattern with no stromal/vascular/pleural invasion.
- They grow along the pre-existing structures without destruction of surrounding alveolar architecture.
  - So, this type of growth pattern has been termed "**lepidic**" growth.

What is the histologic specialty of squamous cell carcinoma?

- Histologically, this tumor is characterized by presence of:
  - Keratinization and/or
  - Intercellular bridges.
- Keratinization occurs in the form of:
  - Squamous pearls (Fig. 9.8)
  - Individual cells with dense eosinophilic cytoplasm.

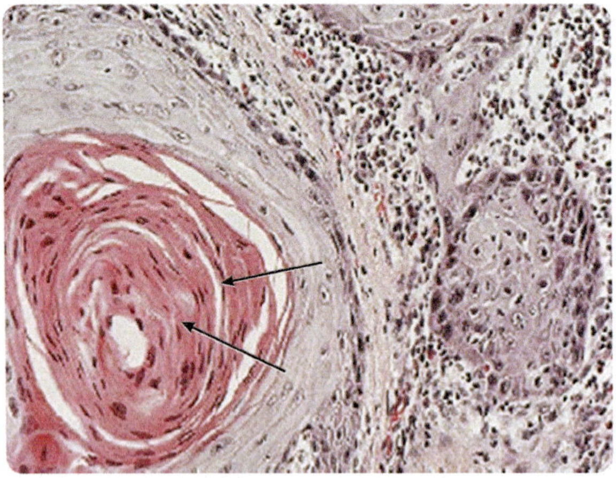

Fig. 9.8: Histological tissue section from a sample of squamous cell carcinoma of lung showing keratin pearls (arrows) formed by layers of keratinization. Reproduced under the permission of National Cancer Institute at National Institute of Health

What is Azzopardi effect?

- It is seen in high grade small cell carcinoma of lung, where necrosis is very common.
- When blood vessels near the tumor is stained with H and E stain, the full thickness of the blood vessel exhibit deeply basophilic staining.
- This occurs due to deposition of DNA and other necrotic materials within the vessel wall.

Which type of lung carcinoma shows highest frequency of p53 mutations?

Squamous cell carcinoma.

Which type of lung carcinoma shows highest frequency of KRAS mutations?

Adenocarcinoma.

What are the anatomic complications caused by lung carcinoma?

1. Emphysema due to partial obstruction of airways.
2. Atelectasis due to total obstruction of airways.
3. Suppurative/ulcerative bronchitis.
4. Bronchiectasis.
5. Lung abscess.
6. Superior vena cava syndrome due to compression of SVC.
7. Pericarditis.
8. Pleuritis.
9. Rib destruction due to chest wall invasion.
10. Horner syndrome due to sympathetic ganglia invasion.

Which histologic variants of lung carcinoma are more associated with paraneoplastic syndromes?

- Small cell carcinomas: ACTH and ADH production.
- Squamous cell carcinomas: Hypercalcemia.

What are the paraneoplastic syndromes caused by lung carcinoma?

The paraneoplastic syndromes caused by lung carcinoma are mainly due to elaboration of various hormones by the carcinoma cells. They are:

Hormones	Paraneoplastic syndromes
ADH	Hyponatremia
ACTH	Cushing's syndrome
PTH	Hypercalcemia
Calcitonin	Hypocalcemia
Gonadotropins	Gynecomastia
Serotonin and bradykinin	Carcinoid syndrome

Bronchiectasis

Description

It is a specimen of cut section of lung with marked dilation of the bronchi and bronchioles with fibrosis in the adjoining areas.

- So, this specimen is identified as "Bronchiectasis" (Fig. 9.9).

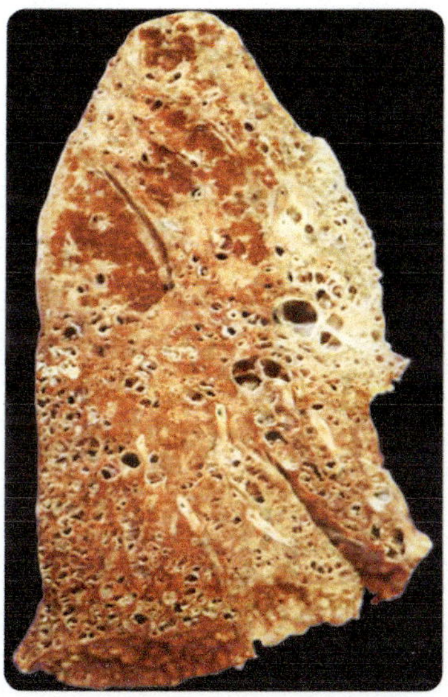

Fig. 9.9: Bronchiectasis. This slice of lung shows extensive, peripheral honeycombing (architectural distortion) in upper and lower lobes. The cystic spaces represent bronchiolectasis. The dark brown areas in the upper lung represent normal lung parenchyma. Reproduced under the permission of Martha L. Warnock, University of California, San Francisco

Define bronchiectasis.

Bronchiectasis is a disease characterized by permanent dilation of bronchi and bronchioles caused by destruction of the muscle and elastic tissue, resulting from a chronic necrotizing infection.

What are the two major pathological points associated with bronchiectasis?

Obstruction and infection.

What are the types of bronchiectasis and what are their causes?

Types	Causes
Obstructive	It occurs by partial/complete obstruction of bronchial lumen by any of the following causative agents: • Neoplasm • Foreign body • Mucus secretion • Lymphadenopathy
Infective/ Inflammatory	It occurs due to repeated episodes of infections. Most common causes are: • Pneumonia • Pertussis Some of the rare causes are: • Kartagener's syndrome • Primary ciliary dyskinesia (These 2 diseases are associated with abnormality in ciliary movements and subsequent accumulation of bacteria)

What are the important features of bronchiectasis?

- They usually affect the lower lobes of the lungs bilaterally.
- The bronchi and bronchioles are extensively dilated.
- The walls of bronchi and bronchioles are intensely inflamed.

- There are areas of desquamation and ulceration of epithelial lining.

What are the complications of bronchiectasis?

1. Hemoptysis
2. Lung abscess
3. Fibrosis
4. Amyloidosis
5. Bronchopleural fistula
6. Squamous metaplasia and squamous cell carcinoma (due to extensive desquamation of the epithelial lining, susceptibility to metaplastic changes increases greatly).

SECTION–II

SLIDES

Pathology Practical Slides Identification

CHAPTER

10

Acute appendicitis

A. Section showing histology of appendix.
B. Lumen is filled up with acute inflammatory infiltrate of neutrophils, macrophages, fibrin, RBC, degenerated epithelial cells, etc.
C. Mucosa—Necrosed and ulcerated.
D. Submucosa and muscle layer—Intense infiltrate of neutrophils and eosinophils (Fig. 10.1).

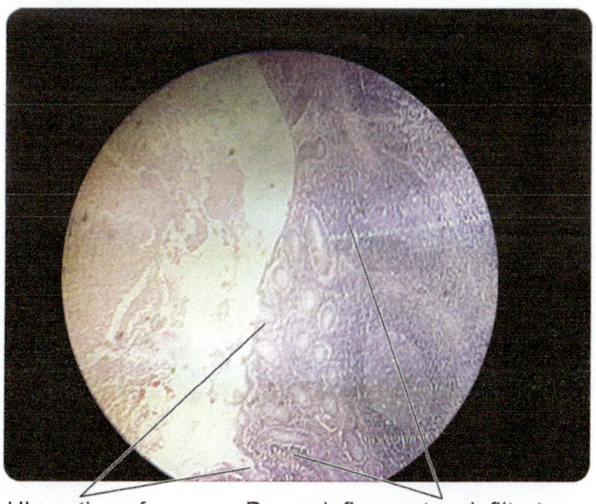

Fig. 10.1: Acute appendicitis

Chronic cholecystitis

A. Section showing histology of gallbladder (absence of submucosa).
B. Mucosa—Ulcerated (Fig. 10.2).

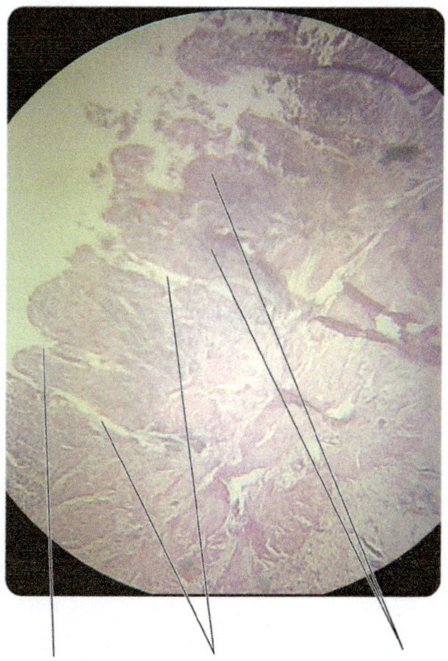

Fig. 10.2: Chronic cholecystitis

C. Dense infiltration of macrophages, lymphocytes and plasma cells.
D. There is presence of RA sinus (Rokitansky-Aschoff sinus) which is formed by invagination of the discontinuous mucous membrane into the muscle layer and forming gland-like structure.

Colloid goiter

A. Section showing histology of thyroid tissue.
B. Glands are dilated and filled up with deeply eosinophilic colloid.
C. Lining epithelial cells are low cuboidal or flattened (Fig. 10.3).

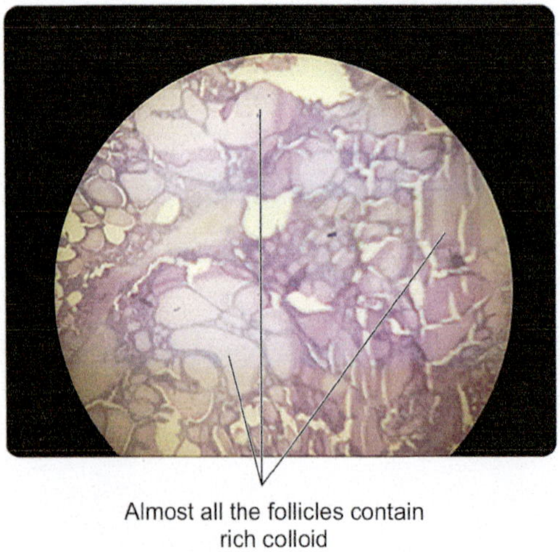

Fig. 10.3: Colloid goiter

Capillary hemangioma

A. Section showing histology of skin.
B. In the deep dermis and subcutaneous layer, there are closely packed blood filled capillaries lined by flattened epithelial cells and separated by scant connective tissue stroma (Fig. 10.4).

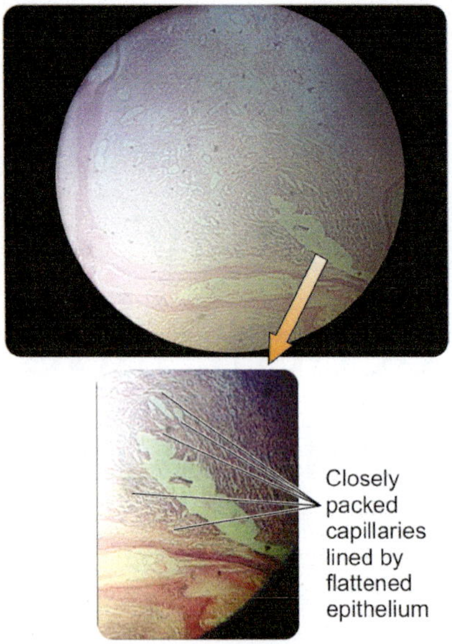

Fig. 10.4: Capillary hemangioma

Cavernous hemangioma

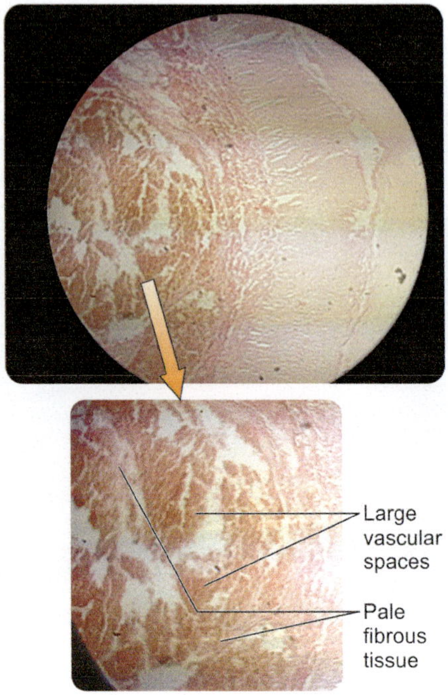

Fig. 10.5: Cavernous hemangioma

A. Section showing a number of large dilated blood filled vascular spaces lined by flattened epithelium (Fig. 10.5).
B. The vascular spaces are separated by modest connective tissue stroma. Intravascular thrombosis is common.

Tuberculosis of lymph node

A. Section showing histology of lymph node.
B. There are areas of granuloma consisting of a granular necrosed material (caseation), surrounded by a zone of epithelioid cells (pale elongated nuclei and abundant pale foamy cytoplasm) along with a few Langhans' giant cells, surrounded by a zone of lymphocytes and that is surrounded by a zone of fibrosis (Fig. 10.6).

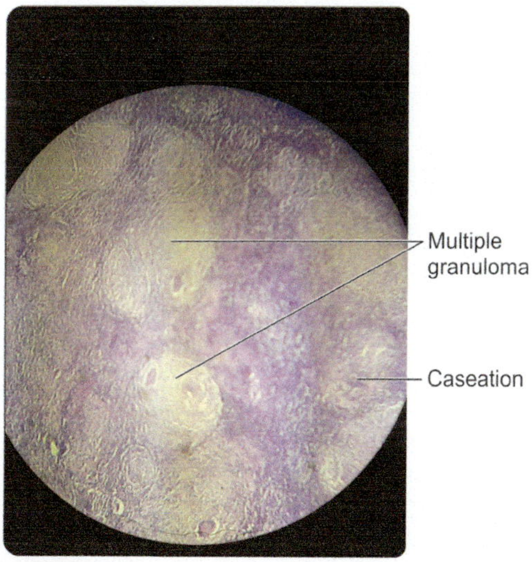

Fig. 10.6: Lymph node TB

Tuberculosis of intestine

A. Section showing histology of intestine.
B. There are areas of granuloma consisting of a granular necrosed material (caseation), surrounded by a zone of epithelioid cells (pale elongated nuclei and abundant pale foamy cytoplasm) along with a few Langhans' giant cells, surrounded by a zone of lymphocytes and that is surrounded by a zone of fibrosis (Fig. 10.7).

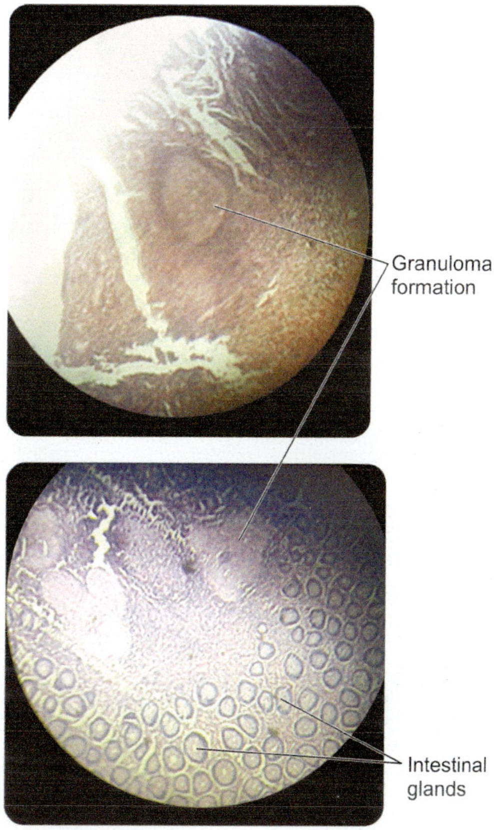

Fig. 10.7:Intestine TB

Adenocarcinoma

A. Section is showing glandular morphology.
B. The submucosa and muscle layers are infiltrated by neoplastic cells having large hyperchromatic nuclei, which are arranges in an acinar pattern (Fig. 10.8).

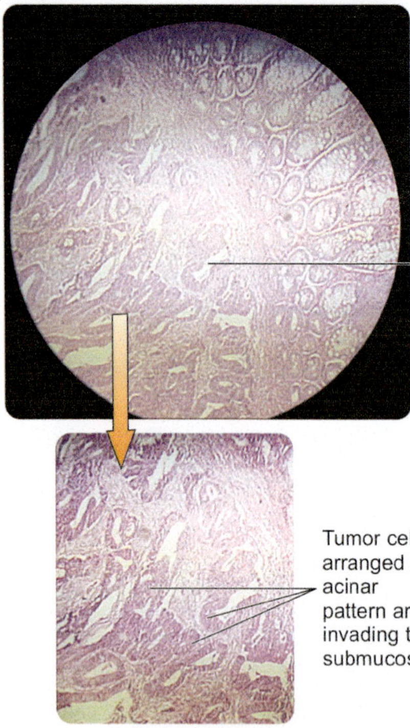

Fig. 10.8: Adenocarcinoma

Secretory endometrium

A. Section showing histology of endometrium.
B. Endometrial glands are tortuous with characteristic *sawtooth appearance* lined by columnar epithelial cells.
C. Lumen of glands containing secretion (Fig. 10.9).

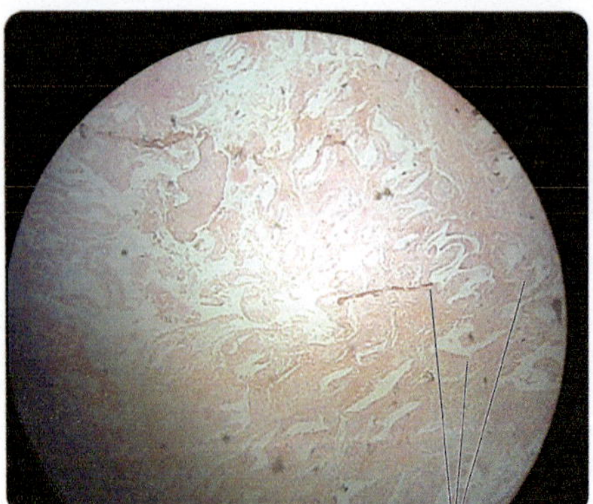

Fig. 10.9: Secretory endometrium

Proliferative endometrium

A. Section showing histology of endometrium.
B. The endometrial glands are more or less uniformly tubular and lined by cuboidal/columnar epithelium.
C. Stroma is compact and cellular (Fig. 10.10).

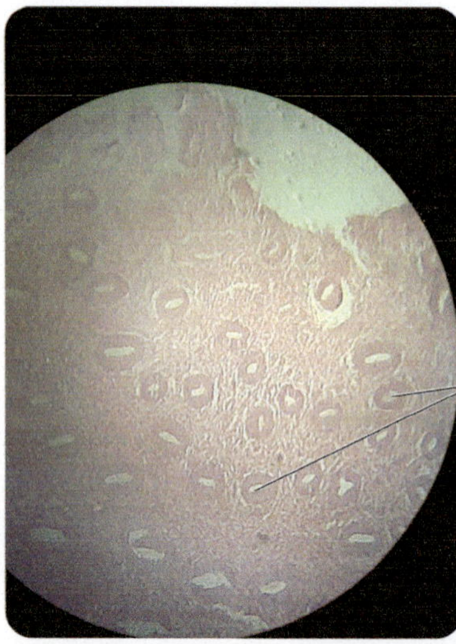

Fig. 10.10:Proliferative endometrium

Benign hypertrophy of prostate (BHP)

A. Section showing histology of prostate (fibromusculoglandular nature).
B. The glands are lined by columnar epithelial cells with uniform basal nuclei and fine granular pale eosinophilic cytoplasm.
C. The gland acini show papillary infolding within the lumen and reddish secretion of the gland, which is called "*Corpora amylacea*" (Fig. 10.11).

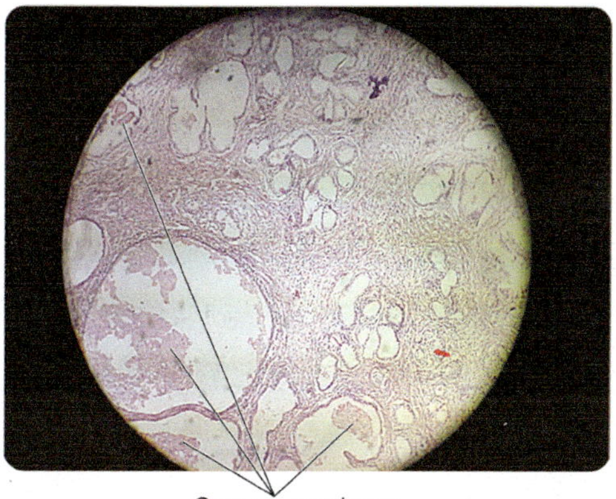

Fig. 10.11: Benign hypertrophy of prostate

Lipoma

A. Section showing histology of a tumor composed of normal looking adipose tissue.
B. The mass of adipose tissue is separated by irregular fibrous septa (Fig. 10.12).

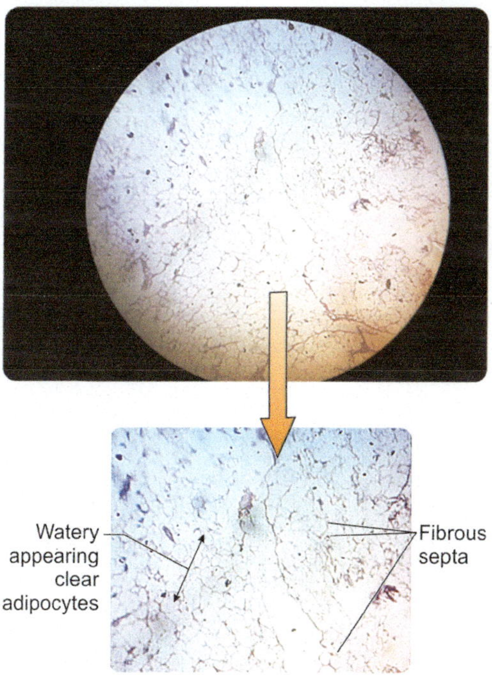

Fig. 10.12: Lipoma

Cirrhosis of liver

A. Section showing histology of liver.
B. Normal architecture is lost.
C. Fibrous band extending from portal tract to central vein and portal tract to portal tract is found.
D. Regenerated nodules (micronodule and macronodules) are found (Fig. 10.13).

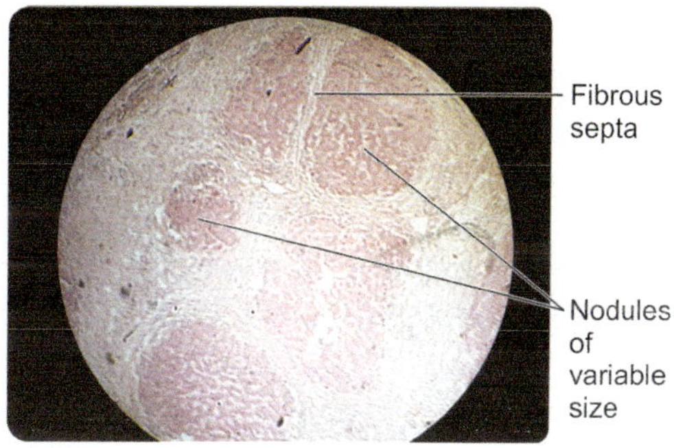

Fig. 10.13: Cirrhosis of liver

Fatty liver

A. Section showing histology of liver.
B. Normal architecture of liver is preserved.

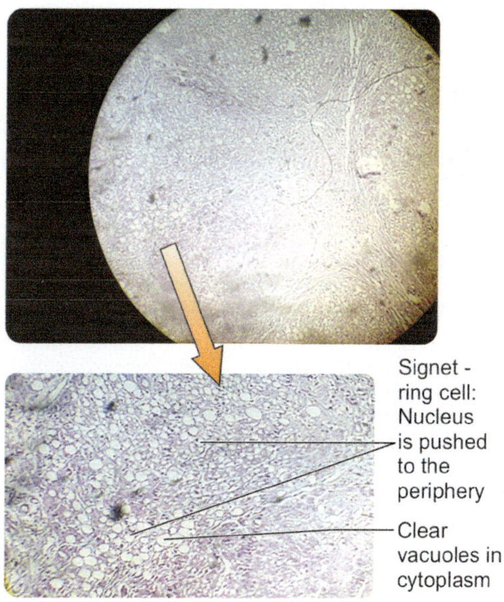

Fig. 10.14: Fatty liver

C. Hepatocytes show large clear vacuoles in cytoplasm.
D. Nucleus has been pushed to the periphery by the cytoplasmic vacuoles; the shape is called "*Signet-ring*" (Fig. 10.14).

Mucinous cystadenoma of ovary

A. Section showing histology of ovary.
B. There are multiple cystic spaces lined by single layer of columnar epithelium.
C. The cystic spaces are separated by fibrovascular stroma and the epithelial cells have uniform basal nuclei and abundant clear cytoplasm (Fig. 10.15).

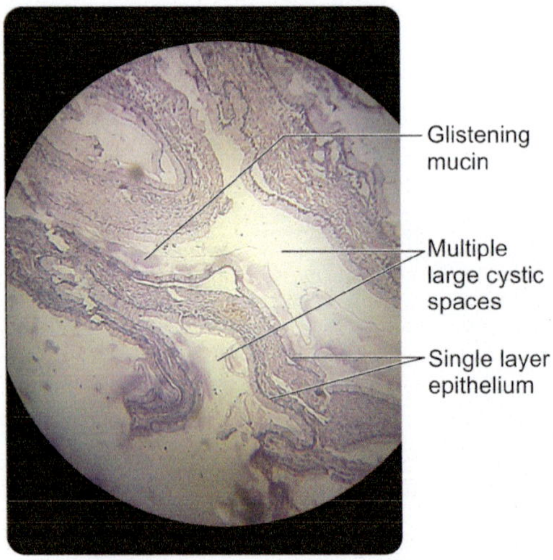

Fig. 10.15: Cystadenoma of ovary

Basal cell carcinoma of skin

A. Section showing histology of skin.
B. The dermis is infiltrated by groups of small basophilic round/fusiform cells having prominent dark-stained nuclei and scanty basophilic cytoplasm, embedded in a mucinous matrix (Fig. 10.16).

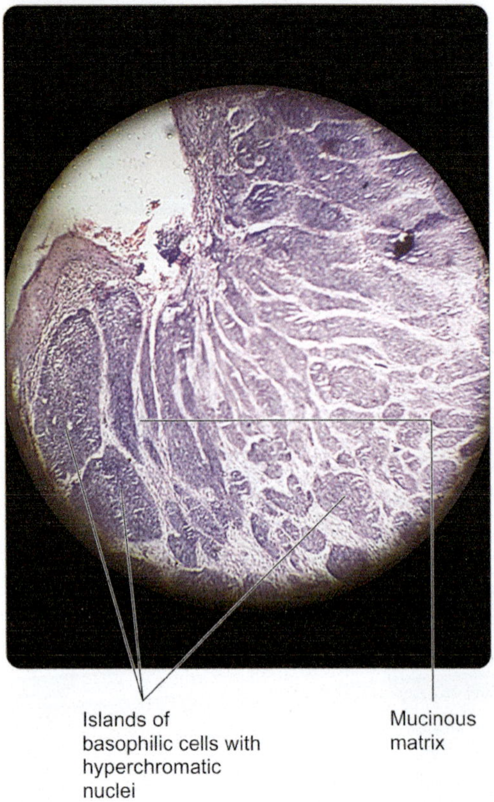

Fig. 10.16: Basal cell carcinoma of skin

Squamous papilloma of skin

A. Section showing histology of skin.
B. Ridges are elongated and bent inward at both the margins of the lesion.
C. There are exophytic papillary projections clothed by thickened epidermis.
D. The papillary processes have a fibrovascular core (Fig. 10.17).

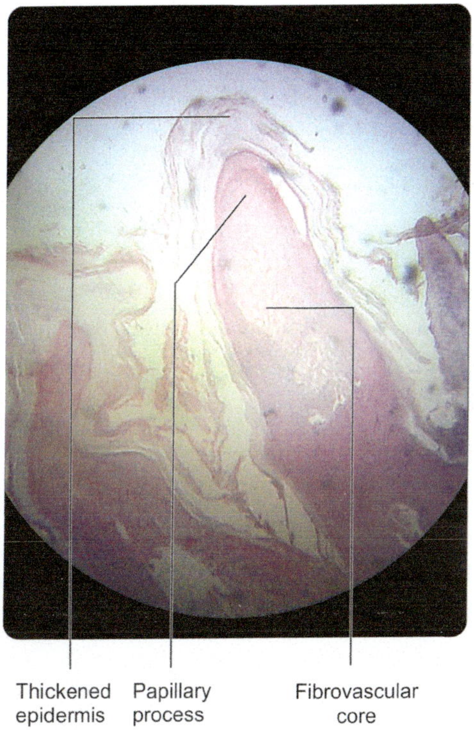

Fig. 10.17: Squamous papilloma of skin

Squamous cell carcinoma of skin

A. Section showing histology of skin.
B. The dermis is invaded by atypical squamous cells having hyperchromatic nuclei.
C. The neoplastic cells show abnormal keratinization in the form of cell nests deep within dermis (Fig. 10.18).

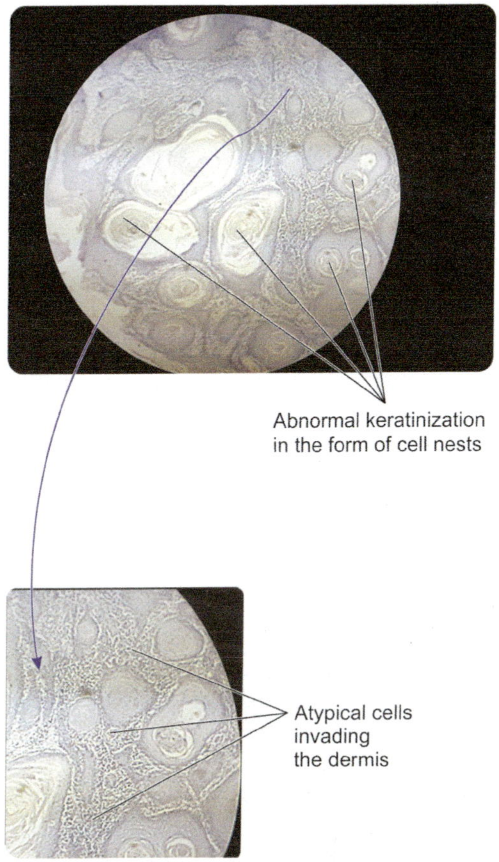

Fig. 10.18: Squamous cell carcinoma of skin

Malignant melanoma of skin

A. Section showing histology of skin.
B. There are clumps of spindle shaped-polyhedral cells with hyperchromatic nuclei.
C. Some of these cells (melanoma cells) contain brownish pigments in the cytoplasm (Fig. 10.19).

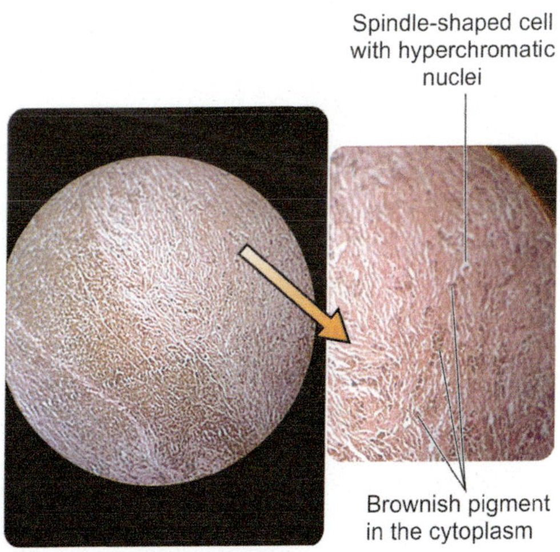

Fig. 10.19: Malignant melanoma of skin

Scirrhous carcinoma of breast

A. Section showing islets of cells having hyperchromatic nuclei and scanty cytoplasm.

B. The groups of neoplastic cells are surrounded by abundant dense fibrous tissue (Fig. 10.20).

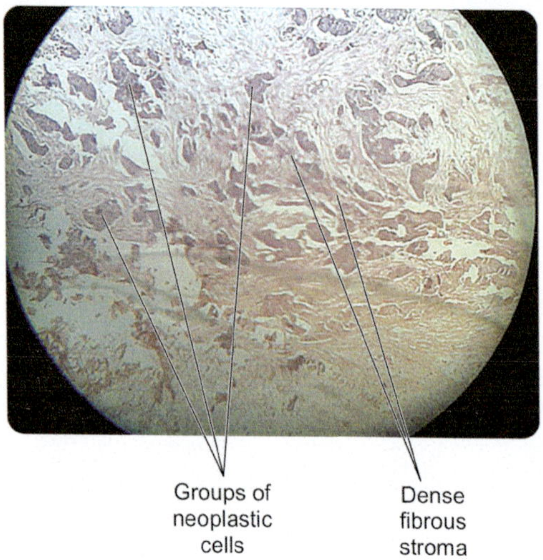

Fig. 10.20: Scirrhous carcinoma of breast

Fibroadenoma of breast

A. Section showing elongated branching compressed mammary ductules.

B. In between the ductules there are abundant pale fibrous tissue/stroma pressing the ductules (Fig. 10.21).

Renal cell carcinoma

A. Section showing histology of kidney.

B. Elsewhere the section shows tumor cells with dark pyknotic nuclei and clear cytoplasm. (possibly clear cell carcinoma)

C. The cells are arranged in sheets and cords with scanty fibrovascular stroma (Fig. 10.22).

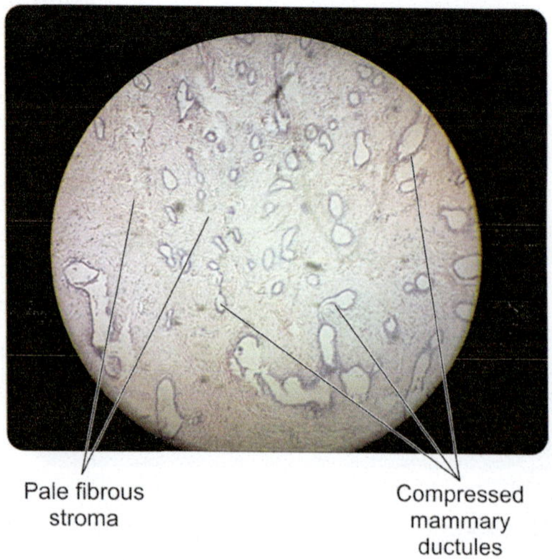

Fig. 10.21: Fibroadenoma of breast

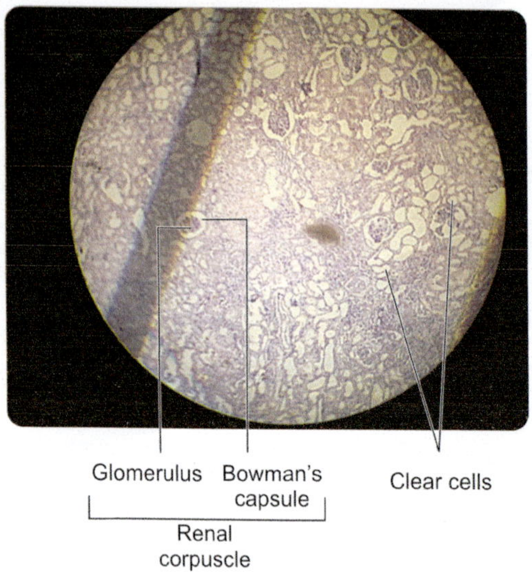

Fig. 10.22: Renal cell carcinoma

Pleomorphic salivary adenoma

A. Section showing histology of a tumor composed of many small glands lined by cuboidal epithelium.
B. The lumen contains eosinophilic secretion.
C. There is abundant myxochondroid stroma (Fig. 10.23).

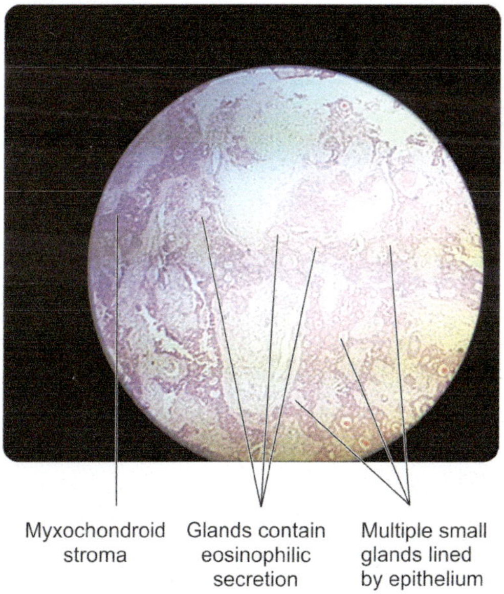

Fig. 10.23: Pleomorphic salivary adenoma

Seminoma testes

A. Section showing histology of a tumor composed of sheets of uniform cells divided into poorly demarcated lobules by delicate fibrous septa with lymphocytic infiltrate.
B. Seminoma cells are large and round, having a large central nucleus and a clear watery cytoplasm.
C. The cytoplasm contains variable amount of glycogen which is washed during slide preparation (Fig. 10.24).

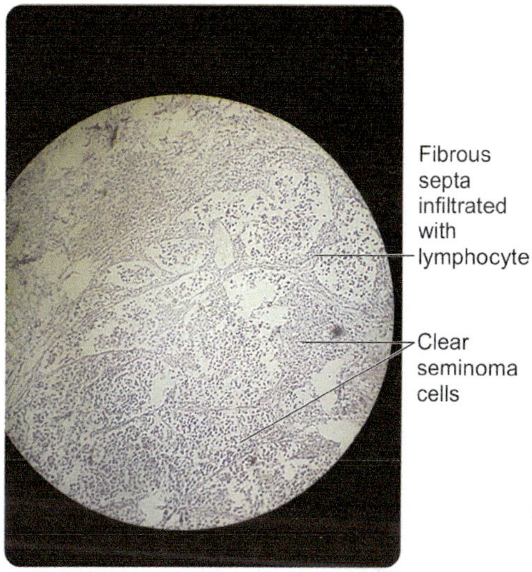

Fig. 10.24: Seminoma testes

Giant cell tumor of bone

A. Section showing histology of tumor containing many osteoclastic giant cells in a background of mononuclear stromal cells.
B. The cells have large number of vesicular nuclei and moderate amount of cytoplasm.
C. There may be areas of hemorrhage and necrosis (Fig. 10.25).

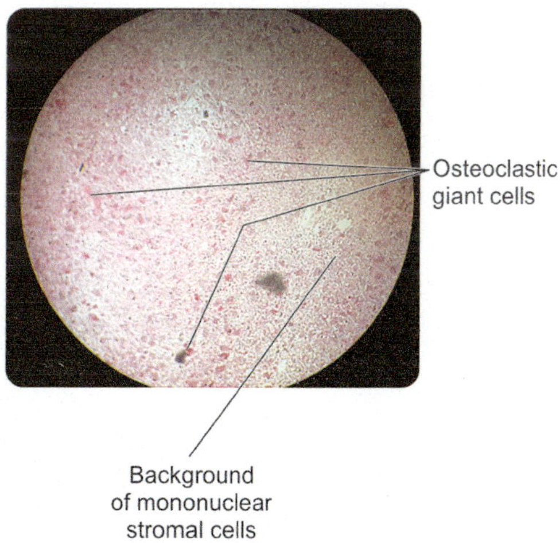

Fig. 10.25: Giant cell tumor of bone

Osteosarcoma

A. Section showing histology of a tumor composed of dark-stained elongated oval pleomorphic cells.
B. They form the dense lace-like pattern of neoplastic bone formation (Fig. 10.26).

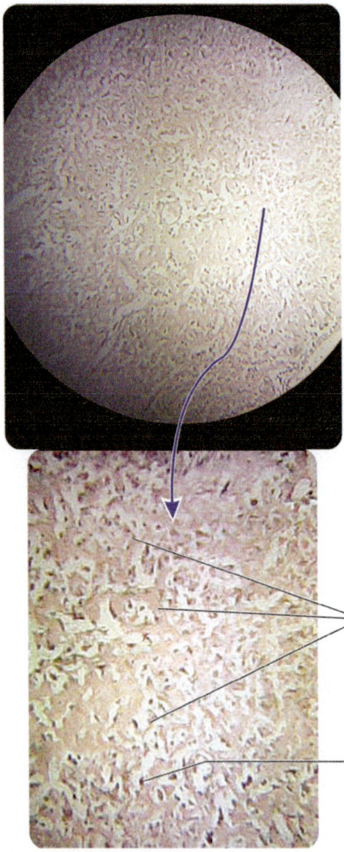

Fig. 10.26: Osteosarcoma

Chronic lymphocytic leukemia (CLL)

- This peripheral blood smear is showing numerous small lymphocytes with condensed chromatin and scant cytoplasm.
- A disrupted tumor cells (smudge cell) is being seen in the center, which is characteristic of CLL.
- Spherocytes (hyperchromatic, round erythrocytes) can also be seen (Fig. 10.27).

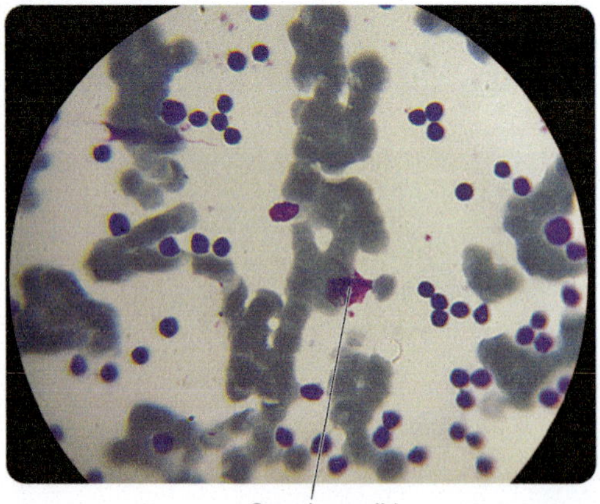

Fig. 10.27: Chronic lymphocytic leukemia

Chronic myeloid leukemia (CML)

- Peripheral blood smear is showing numerous mature neutrophils and some metamyelocytes (Fig. 10.28).

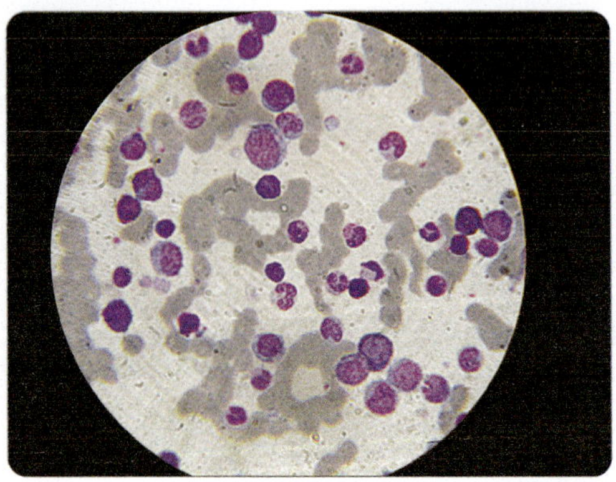

Fig. 10.28: Chronic myeloid leukemia

Bibliography

1. Bailey, Love. A Short Textbook of Surgery, 25th ed.
2. Brunicardi CS. Schwartz's Principles of Surgery, 9th ed.
3. Essential Orthopaedics, 4th ed. Maheshwari.
4. Faust T, Reddy KR. The Clinician's Guide to Liver Disease.
5. Guidelines on Renal Cell Carcinoma by European Association of Urology, April 2010.
6. Huckstep RL. Typhoid fever and other salmonella infections. Edinburgh, E and S. Livingstone Ltd, 1962.
7. Kleiner DE, Brunt EM, Van Natta M, Behling C, Contos MJ, Cummings OW, Ferrell LD, Liu YC, Torbenson MS, Unalp-Arida A, Yeh M, McCullough AJ, Sanyal AJ. Nonalcoholic Steatohepatitis Clinical Research Network. Design and validation of a histological scoring system for nonalcoholic fatty liver disease. Hepatology. 2005 June;41(6):1313–21.
8. Park's Textbook of Community Medicine, 22nd ed.
9. Rheumatic fever and Rheumatic heart disease: Report of a WHO expert consultation: 29th October- 1st November, 2001.
10. Robbins, Cotran: Pathologic Basis of Disease, 8th ed.

Index

Page numbers followed by *f* refer to figure and *t* refer to table

L

M

N

O

P

Q

R

S

T

U

V